**DISCLAIMER AND TERMS OF USE AGREEMENT:**

**(Please Read This Before Using This Book)**

This information is not presented by a medical practitioner and is for educational and informational purposes only. The content is not intended to be a substitute for professional medical advice, diagnosis, or treatment. Always seek the advice of your physician or other qualified health provider with any questions you may have regarding a medical condition. Never disregard professional medical advice or delay in seeking it because of something you have read.

Since natural and/or dietary supplements are not FDA approved, they must be accompanied by a two-part disclaimer on the product label: that the statement has not been evaluated by FDA and that the product is not intended to "diagnose, treat, cure or prevent any disease.

The author and publisher of this course and the accompanying materials have used their best efforts in preparing this course. The author and publisher make no representation or warranties with respect to the accuracy, applicability, fitness, or completeness of the contents of this course. The information contained in this course is strictly for educational purposes. Therefore, if you wish to apply ideas contained in this course, you are taking full responsibility for your actions.

The author and publisher disclaim any warranties (express or implied), merchantability, or fitness for any particular purpose. The author and publisher shall in no event be held liable to any party for any direct, indirect, punitive, special, incidental or other consequential damages arising directly or indirectly from any use of this material, which is provided "as is", and without warranties.

As always, the advice of a competent legal, tax, accounting, medical or other professional should be sought. The author and publisher do not warrant the performance, effectiveness or applicability of any sites listed or linked to in this course.

All links are for information purposes only and are not warranted for content, accuracy or any other implied or explicit purpose.



# Read all my books on Kindle for free without downloading except you want to buy them.

# Contents

# Causes Of Back Pain

Back pain will inhibit millions of Americans this year, and an estimated 80% of us will experience back pain sometime in our lives. For some, the pain can be excruciating. Back pain can be caused by a large number of injuries or conditions, thus making a proper diagnosis both difficult and critical. Back pain that occurs with other symptoms like fever and chills, severe abdominal pain or bladder and bowel problems can be an indication of a serious medical condition, and should be evaluated by your doctor immediately.

Musculoskeletal strains are more common among people who live sedentary lifestyles. Those with a higher level of physical fitness generally have stronger muscles in the back, legs and abdomen, all of which help support the back. Perhaps the most significant risk factor is obesity. The strain of carrying excess weight can contribute greatly to back pain. Regular exercise and a balanced diet can help control obesity, and reduce the frequency of back pain episodes.

There are many conditions that can cause back pain other than musculoskeletal strains. They include:

- Arthritis, a disease that causes inflammation of the joints. Three types of arthritis that affect the spine are osteoarthritis, rheumatoid arthritis and ankolyzing spondylitis.
- A herniated disc, or ruptured disc, occurs when the hard outer coating of the discs, the circular pieces of connective tissue that cushion the vertebrae, are damaged. These discs may leak, irritating nearby nerves. A herniated disk can cause severe sciatica, nerve pain that radiates down the leg.
- Spinal stenosis is a condition where the spinal canal narrows, compressing the nerves inside. It is often caused by bone spurs which are a result of osteoarthritis. Compression of the nerves can lead to pain, numbness in the legs and the loss of bladder or bowel control.
- Spondylolisthesis is a condition where a vertebra of the slips out of place. As the spine tries to stabilize itself, the joints between the slipped vertebra and adjacent vertebrae can become enlarged. This can pinch nerves, causing low back pain and severe sciatica leg pain.
- Vertebral fractures can be caused by trauma or by osteoporosis, a disease where the bones become fragile.
- Degenerative disc disease is an aging process where the discs between the vertebrae break down over time.

# How To Prevent Back Pain

Simple lower back pain can be caused by straining the muscles, tendon or ligaments of the lower back. The most effective prevention is to take care as to how you lift heavy objects. Do not try to lift any significant weight by bending over the object. You should bend your knees and then lift with your legs. Avoid twisting your body while lifting. When moving heavy objects, pushing is less stressful than pulling. Routine activities, such as housework or gardening, can cause back pain. Avoid standing flat-footed while bent over.

A sedentary lifestyle will contribute to back problems.

Regular exercise will improve the flexibility and strength of the muscles which support your lower back. These include the abdominal muscles, as well as those in the legs and back. A simple exercise routine can help prevent back pain throughout your life. Obesity is a common cause of back pain. Aerobic exercise can help manage weight concerns. Swimming, jogging or even walking are all activities that will help you lose weight and feel better.

In addition to exercise, a proper diet is essential in managing your weight. However, there are also two nutrients, calcium and vitamin D, that help build healthy and strong bones and prevent osteoporosis, which can cause bone fractures that lead to back pain.

Many people whose jobs involve sitting for long periods of time experience back pain. It is important to get up and move around regularly. If driving for long periods of time, take the time to stop and get out of your vehicle.

Stretching your muscles and improving blood flow to your lower body will help prevent back pain, as well as help keep you alert for the rest of your trip.

Changing the position in which you sleep can also help prevent back pain. The best positions are either to sleep lying on your side with your legs bent, or lying on your back with a pillow under your knees. A firm mattress is usually the best bet. A sheet of plywood can be placed between the box spring and the mattress in order to increase the firmness of your bed.

## <u>Non-Surgical Treatment For Back Pain</u>

Back pain may be relieved with a variety of techniques. For most common occurrences of back pain, a regiment of rest, hot and cold compresses, exercise and therapy, as well as various pain medications can be used to reduce the pain and provide a level of comfort.

Hot and cold compresses, used separately or by alternating, can have great benefit in reducing back pain. Heat is used to relax the muscles. It works by dilating the blood vessels, which improves the flow of oxygen to the affected area and reduces pain and muscle spasms. Cold packs are used to reduce inflammation, such as that from arthritis or injury. This works by decreasing the size of blood vessels and the flow of blood to the area. It is important to avoid prolonged application of either heat or cold packs, especially near the organs found in the abdominal cavity.

Exercising is of great benefit both to someone suffering from back pain and for anyone hoping to avoid it in the future. If you are suffering from acute back pain, exercising may not be possible or even a good idea.

However, for chronic back pain, a regular exercise program is recommended. Exercises will help strengthen the muscles that support the back, and increase flexibility and range of motion. A physical therapist can help you in developing an exercise plan that is suitable for you and your condition.

Nonprescription medicines can be used to reduce pain. They include medications like aspirin Tylenol, which are meant for general pain relief. Anti-inflammatory drugs are used to reduce swelling. These include such nonprescription medications as ibuprofen (Motrin, Advil). Stronger prescription-based medication is available, both as pain relievers and anti-inflammatories.

## Surgical Treatments For Back Pain

While the majority of treatment for lower back pain is non-surgical, there are some conditions for which surgery is appropriate. As well, in some rare cases, surgery can be used to treat chronic back pain for which other treatments have failed.

In a laminectomy, part of the lamina, a portion of the bone on the back of the vertebrae, is removed. It can be used to treat herniated discs and spinal stenosis. In microdiscectomy a much smaller incision is made and the doctor uses a magnifying lens to locate the disc.

The smaller incision may reduce pain and the disruption of tissues, and it reduces the size of the surgical scar.

With a laser discectomy, a laser is used to vaporize the tissue in the disc, reducing its size and relieving pressure on the nerves.

Spinal fusion may be used to treat spondylolisthesis and degenerative disc disease. In spinal fusion, two or more vertebrae are joined together using bone grafts, screws, and rods. The fused area of the spine becomes immobilized.

Vertebral fractures can be caused by trauma or by osteoporosis. A vertebroplasty injects a cement-like mixture called polymethyacrylate into the fractured vertebra to stabilize the spine. Kyphoplasty inserts a balloon device to help restore the height and shape of the spine before injecting polymethyacrylate to repair the fractured vertebra.

Disc replacement surgery can now be done in cases where the disc is severely damaged. Here the disc is simply removed and replaced with a synthetic disc.

# Alternative Treatments For Back Pain

The term alternative therapy covers a wide array of treatments, with a corresponding variation in levels of acceptance amongst the medical community.

Alternative medicine is a growing field, but sometimes relies more on anecdotal evidence than careful study.

The most reputable alternative treatments include chiropractic, prolotherapy, acupuncture and acupressure, and massage therapy.

Chiropractors use spinal manipulation to adjust the spine. Their goal is to ease pressure on the nervous system by properly aligning the spine. Spinal manipulation tries to restore joint mobility by applying a controlled force into joints that have become restricted in their movement. Chiropractic is the most popular form of alternative therapy.

Prolotherapy is a treatment in which a sugar solution or other irritating substance is injected into the periosteum, the fibrous tissue covering the bones, in order to strengthen the attachment of tendons and ligaments.

Acupuncture and acupressure are based on the ancient Chinese philosophy that a life force called Qi flows through the body. If the flow is impeded, the body can become ill. Acupuncture uses needles to unblock the flow of Qi, while acupressure uses massage to accomplish the same thing.

Massage therapy can benefit back pain sufferers by increasing blood flow and circulation, decreasing tension in the muscles, reducing pain caused by tight muscles and even improving sleep. Massage therapy can provide relief for many common conditions that cause back pain, such as arthritis, fibromyalgia, sports injuries and various other soft tissue sprains and strains.

# Exercise For Back Pain: Mattresses

Night time is a period when we all want to relax from our everyday tensions and troubles of life. However, if this also turns out to be a discomforting experience, there cannot be anything more annoying. We all want to stay comfortable in our cocoons at night, but money is also an important consideration.

Due to this, homeowners have been divided into two divisions – ones who are ready to spend any price for their comfort and the others who are quite economical and therefore not very choosy about the mattress they are using unless they can actually afford those expensive comforts of luxurious mattresses.

**Memory foam mattresses – a remedy for your back pain**
The good news especially for these economical homeowners is that superior memory foam mattresses are now accessible at affordable rates providing you a refreshing and relaxed sleep.

One of the most common complaints that people make relating to their sleep is about their back pain. People are more likely to change sides frequently during the sleep if their hips or back is getting hurt. Foam mattresses cushion the body so well that you do not feel any pain and ensures you a sound sleep.

Even when you have any temporary pains like pregnancy, upgrading to this fine quality mattress can provide you with great rest.

By enhancing your experience of sleep, it can help you to rest your body and thereby increase your energy levels, so that you achieve more than what you decide without feeling lethargic. The popularity of memory foam mattresses has increased tremendously in the past few years. Also, its price is dropping with every passing year.

**Regular v/s memory foam mattress**
The disparity that lies between any regular mattress and memory foam mattress is awesome. They don't only have a visual appeal, they are something that you should actually go to the sales floor and feel it yourself to realize its true worth. Though most manufacturers make

available a complimentary trial period for these mattresses, but it is hardly possible to return it back after the trial period once you have experienced the luxury of sleeping on them.

## Upgrade gradually to mattress

In case, you don't want to invest straightway into the memory foam mattress, you can initiate with a memory foam pillow or a topper. This will gradually acquaint you with the benefits of these luxurious products. It is advisable to start with a topper only and then shift to the mattress to make your experience the most contented one.

# Exercise For Back Pain: Avoiding Back Pain In Pregnancy

Lower back pain is a complaint that most women yell about in the initial stages of pregnancy. At this time, the abdomen expands and it pulls the lower back forward.

Hormones are responsible to relax muscles and joints in the entire body. This puts a lot of pressure on the back, causing pain. Reading further will provide you with some tips that can help you to reduce your lower back pain during pregnancy.

**Tips to get rid of lower back pain in early pregnancy**

- *Right posture -* The foremost thing that you should mind to reduce your lower back pain is to uphold the right posture. You should always stand and sit straight with your shoulders held back. Make sure that you do not get stained by your abdomen pulling forward your lower back.

If your work requires you to sit a lot, choose a chair that supports your back. Do not sit cross-legged and often take s small walk to stretch yourself.

- *Body pillow -* Remember not to lie on the back while sleeping; rather try to be on your sides. You can keep a body pillow for support under the abdomen and amongst your knees for complete support. This will reduce pressure from your back and keep the body in good posture or alignment.

- *Diet* – Eat healthy and nutritious food that is good both for you and your baby's health. Be cautious about gaining too much of weight, as it is harmful for both of you and will also put a strain on your back all the more. You can also try some exercises after consulting your doctor.

- *Shoes* – Wear low-heeled footwear that is comfortable. High-heeled shoes increase the pressure on your back and also increase the possibility of falling.

- *Massage* – If you are unable to bear the pain, chiropractic care and massage are the options that you can try. Massaging with heated oils on the affected area can also be of great help. Do not take any of these treatments without consultation with your doctor.

**How To Win Your War Against Back Pain**

Acetaminophen can also be taken for pain relief at the time of pregnancy. Consuming NSAIDS like Advil, Motrin and many other kinds of ibuprofen is not very safe at this time.

- *Lift* – Be careful not to lift anything by bending over your waist or heavy objects on your head. Try to keep your back as straight as possible.

Be sure that your doctor is aware of any kind of back pains that you may be suffering from as it may also be an indication for premature labor that may require immediate attention. No doubt, pregnancy is accompanied with a lot of pains, but at last with a new born in your hand its worth it all.

# Exercise For Back Pain: Learning From Videos

It is essential for you to learn things with great care when you gain knowledge by looking at an instructional video as pain in your back can create a real problem for you.

Your back and muscles will become strong with the passage of time if you follow the instructions of the instructional video. In this way you will be able to manage your anxiety on daily basis. The Instructional videos' are a key for learning suitable back exercises.

There are many resolutions and cares for back pain and it may happen to anyone and problems can take place. Thus it is necessary if you are suffering from back pain due to many reasons or if you have received back injuries at your work place which can become the reason of back pain.

## Prevention Is Better Than Cure

There are many ways for that provides avoidance tips for backache. The most suitable method to know about back safety and the avoidance of problems related to back is to see video related to it. The most suitable method to get rid of back pain is having a regular back exercise.

The exercises, which are done, to get rid of pain can also be done for prevention of pain. A suitable instructional video will contain all the information. On some occasions physiotherapy and going to gym may be costly and may also be far away from your home.

## Taking Help From Video

Sometimes it is good for you to buy an instructional video and practice back exercises at home. You can search a suitable instructional video for you with the suggestion of doctor and friends. Your physician can advice you on some specific matters which you need to do in a different manner than an instructional video.

It is mainly important when you are suffering from problems such as asthma, heart attack, or you are elderly, or shapeless then you need to be very careful when you do exercise. It is mainly important that the injury is not getting worse or the exercises are not done properly and not created other problems.

**How To Win Your War Against Back Pain**

The daily suggestion that a back instructional video can recommend besides the regular exercise are standing, walking and sitting with a good posture, bending from the knees and not from the back, not bending too much to pick things up, and use changing sleeping positions. All these activities help in relieving your back pain.

# Exercise For Back Pain: Treatments

It is expected that any kind of pain in back is a serious problem, which can affect about 80% of the population. Many people suffer from serious back pain, which can go in a few days or weeks. There are several remedies, which can begin with simple pain relievers and physical therapy to surgery for critical back problems.

## The Optional Treatment For Back Pain

Many patients are going to have an optional treatment instead of the traditional methods, as they are easy and cost-effective. These methods are beneficial in treating the distress, saving the patient from undergoing medical examinations and unnecessary surgery. This can finally save a lot of money, which is spent on medical bills and health, care costs.

There is one natural treatment for alternative back pain. The examples of some of the alternative treatment methods are as follows:

*Acupuncture:* Acupuncture needles are placed in a pathway where one feels pain on the back. The needles release the blocked energy from affected areas. In a latest survey on 150 patients suffering from back pain, the patients, which had acupuncture over traditional methods, become pain free much faster and for long time.

*Capsaicin Cream:* This is the content one can find in chili peppers. It is very efficient when massage on the distraught area four times in a day. One can get it at health food stores, medical stores and online.

*Vitamin D:* Vitamin D is essential for healthy bones and muscles. A shortage on Vitamin D can become reason of chronic muscle pain in your back. Milk, fish and cereal are good sources of vitamin D.

*Music Therapy:* Music Therapy has proven most beneficial as well as a depression reducer among people who suffer with chronic back pain. The practice of listening to soft music will reduce stress and depression and these are related to chronic backache.

## How To Win Your War Against Back Pain

*Vitamin B-12:* Vitamin B-12 is also vitamin, which is very effective for reducing pain in back. The dairy products and meat are very good sources for Vitamin B-12.

*Magnesium:* Magnesium is very essential for muscle growth, healthy bones as well as provides a very good immune system for just a few of the advantages of mineral. Magnesium rich foods are green vegetables such as spinach, whole grain breads, nuts and bananas.

The other methods to work on pain in the back are yoga; willow bark and Bowen therapy. Each of these treatments takes its own time to treat the backache.

# Exercise For Back Pain: Back Pain Constipation

The back pain constipation is generally found in the adults and is very common these days. There is no need to introduce constipation, which is the major cause of restlessness in the body. The back pain constipation is caused due to chronic constipation. The location of the intestine, as situated near the lower back, results in the back pain due to difficulty in passing the stool.

## What Causes Back pain Constipation?

The studies have shown that the maximum number of people visiting the doctor consists of those, who suffer from the back pain. The back pain occurs in most of the adults due to a number of reasons. The lower back present in the human body is under constant stress due to a number of activities like walking, standing and sitting for a long period.

These reasons add up to the main reason for back pain constipation that is incidence constipation. In addition, if you face difficulty in passing stools out of the body, this also leads to back pain constipation. In the process of passing stools, the sensitive tissues of anus get swollen due to the large amount of pressure employed in the process. The result is often the back pain constipation.

The back pain constipation is also found in the small children. It has been observed that people visiting the physician with the problem of back pain often end up in getting treated for constipation. The most acute effect of back pain constipation is the weakening of the muscles associated with lower back.

## Analyzing The Symptoms

The most significant symptoms of back pain constipation includes:

- Acute pain in the lower back of the body
- Accompanying of stool passing with pain
- Movement of pain from lower back to some areas of torso
- Increase in the pain with passage of time
- Feeling of sickness and decrease in the appetite
- Weakness in the joints of lower body
- Difficulty in passing the tools

**How To Win Your War Against Back Pain**

**Carrying Out the Right Treatment**

There are various methods of treating back pain constipation. The consumption of painkillers and laxatives is the most common one. Some of the physicians also recommend thyroxin as the part of treatment.

The diet plays an important role in treating the back pain constipation. The diet must consist of right quantity of All-Bran along with oat bran. Also, the green vegetables and a lot of water are also helpful in relieving the pain caused due to constipation.

# Advice For How To Get Rid Of Back Pain Now And Later

Since four out of five of us are going to suffer from back pain at one time or another, according to numerous studies, it only makes sense to learn how you can cope with the pain as well as prevent it from happening in the first place.

Though there are some cases of back pain that you can't control – accidents, traumas, pregnancy, etc. – most cases of back pain are related to the way we move and interact with the world around us.

So, if we change the way we move, we can reduce our chances of being sidelined by back pain. Here are some helpful tips that can both help you prevent back pain from being a problem, while also helping you reduce back pain if you've already begun to feel a twinge.

**NOTE:** If you are currently suffering from back pain and any of these tips make the pain worse, stop what you are doing and check with your doctor for further guidance.

**Stand Up Straight**

While most of us realize that we should be correcting our posture more, it's an essential step in preventing and reducing back pain.

Our spines are meant to be in a naturally curved position, but we need to hold our bodies in a certain manner in order to allow the body to sit in this proper position.

When you slouch, the vertebrae in your spine have more pressure put on them, causing pain and possible spinal damage when you continue to slouch throughout your life.

Here is how you can begin to stand up straight:

- Stand with your feet slightly apart, about hip's distance is comfortable for most people.

- Hold your head up high with your gaze forward.

**How To Win Your War Against Back Pain**

- Pull your chin up so that it is parallel with the floor.

- Roll your shoulders slightly back.

- Keep a slight bend in your knees, softening them.

- Put your arms to your sides, with palms facing inward.

- Bring your chest up, as though you were taking a deep breath.

You should be able to draw a line from your ear to the shoulder to your hip to your knee if you are standing up properly.

But the immediate effect will be that your body should feel more relaxed and your neck and back should loosen up.

You can also use these tips when you are sitting down, though your feet should be flat on the floor and knees bent at a ninety degree angle from your chair.

The more you practice this good posture, the more natural it will become

# Head To The Gym

Since your back and neck are supported by the muscles in your body, it only makes sense that the stronger those muscles are, the more likely they will support your body and prevent back and neck pain.

To support your lower back, you will want to focus on abdominal training. A simple abdominal workout should include exercises for each of the major muscle groups:

## Upper Abs – Basic crunches

- Lay on your back with your hands crossed on your chest.
- Place your feet flat on the floor with your knees bent.
- Slowly lift your chest up toward the ceiling, keeping your chin pointed to the ceiling.
- Lift a few inches from the ground, hold for a second and then lower slowly to the ground.

## Lower Abs – Reverse crunches

- Lay on your back your arms at your sides
- Lift your legs up with your knees bent and feet off the floor
- Focusing on your lower abs, lift your buttocks off the floor slowly, keeping the rest of your body in place
- Slowly lower down

## Oblique Muscles – Side crunches

- Lay on your right side with your knees bent
- Support your head with your right arm and bring the left hand to your head
- Crunch toward your legs with the left leg, using the left elbow to guide the movement, lower down.
- Switch sides

**How To Win Your War Against Back Pain**

You can repeat these exercises daily or every other day to help increase your abdominal strength and thus reduce your back pain.

**The More Walking the Better**

One of the best exercises for a healthy back and neck is to get outside and walk more.

Because our bodies fall into a more natural posture when we walk, this will help you strengthen your entire body and allow for better support of any weaker muscles in your core.

Try walking the recommended 10,000 steps a day by purchasing a pedometer and charting your progress. The more active you are, the more strength you are providing to your back – and those are all steps in the right direction.

# When Lifting And Moving Heavy Objects

Many of us have hurt our backs when we were lifting or moving something that was heavier than our muscles were accustomed to. We inadvertently strained our muscles, which can take a long time to heal if the injury was severe enough.

But there are ways we can prevent these kinds of injuries in the future:

- ***Always lift with your knees*** – Instead of thinking of lifting things with your arms and your upper body, focus on your knees and legs when you lift something heavy. The larger muscles in your lower body can more easily adapt to heavier weights.

- ***Be sure to push instead of pull*** – If you have to move something that's heavy, be sure to push the object (if you can) instead of pull it. Because pushing uses more lower body strength, you will reduce the stress on your back and neck.

- ***Hold in your abdominals*** – Whenever you are lifting or moving something, be sure to pull in your abdominal muscles to protect your back. It will help if you take in a deep breath as you do so.

- ***Get help*** – Instead of lifting something that you shouldn't be lifting, maybe you should ask a friend to help you lighten the weight on your back and your body.

- ***Avoid twisting as you lift*** – When lifting something heavy, be sure to move up and down in a straight line. This will help you protect the smaller muscles and ligaments in your back.

- ***Hold the object close you*** – Instead of holding something far away, be sure to hold the item closer to your body, it helps to create a healthier balance.

- ***Never lift anything above shoulder level*** – You aren't as balanced at this height and you can cause a lot of damage to your back.

As you decide that you need to move something heavier, you need to create a plan for how you will move it BEFORE you start to lift.  This will help you plan for any troubles and decide whether you need to enlist more help than you might have on hand.

# <u>Try Drinking More Water</u>

Though the benefits of water have been touted for everything from weight loss to boosting your immune system, water can also help you prevent back pain.

Because the muscles of the body require water in order to function at their highest capacity, you need to make sure you are preventing dehydration from happening.

But the amount of water you need will vary from person to person. Those who are larger in size and who have more muscles will require more water to function properly. Those who are smaller will not need as much water in their bodies.

There are a few easy ways to tell if you are drinking enough water:

- You aren't thirsty
- Your lips aren't dry or chapped
- Your urine is a pale yellow
- You are urinating every two hours

You can drink plain water to help boost your hydration, but you can also choose from the many caffeine free drinks that are available too – juices, decaffeinated coffee, etc.

Certain foods also contain a large amount of water (watermelon, cucumbers, and corn), so these will also count toward your levels of hydration.

# Yoga Can Help

It seems like everyone has tried yoga at one point or another, but can it really help you with back pain?

Here are a few simple postures that you can try at home to help you reduce your current back pain as well as to prevent it from coming back:

- Sit in a chair with your feet on the ground, looking forward. Slowly turn your upper body to one side, using your hands on the side of the chair or the arm rest to guide the movement. The movement should be small and your lower body should not move. Switch sides.

- Lay down with your legs up in the air and against the wall. If this puts too much pressure on your back, you can place a rolled up yoga mat or towel under your lower back for support. Raise your arms over your head and on the floor behind you.

- Lay on the floor with your head supported by towels, your palms up and your shoulder blades flat on the ground. Close your eyes and relax your muscles, allowing your legs to fall apart and your hips to turn outward.

- Sit with your legs out in front of you, legs together. Try to reach up to the ceiling and then down to your toes to provide a deep stretch in your lower back and hips. Slowly bring your self back up to sitting by tightening your abdominal muscles.

There are a number of helpful yoga DVDs and classes available to help you learn the basics of this ancient practice. By helping you focus your breathing and strengthening your core, you can increase the pain free days in your life.

# Foot Massage Tricks

Acupressure and massage are often used to help those with back and neck pain, but even foot massage can help you reduce your pain as well.

Reflexology techniques work on the idea that certain points of the body are related to other parts of the body. The system uses maps that pinpoint areas that you can press in order to release tension in other parts of the body – like the back.

At the end of the day, try some of these techniques for preventing back pain:

- Take one foot in your hand and push along the inner part of the big toenail bed. The other hand should be supporting the big toe as you do this to stabilize the movement. Rotate your finger on this area in a clockwise pattern a few times and then the opposite direction a few times. Switch feet and repeat.
- Move down the foot to the joint of the big toe and rub the outside of this joint in small circles. Switch feet.
- Move toward the outside of the foot where the little toe is and pinch the skin between the bottom of the foot and the bottom of the little toe.  Push into this area in a circular motion, switch directions and then switch feet.

These techniques are for helping back pain once it's already started:

- Have someone hold onto your foot's heel and then have them push alongside the bottom of your foot where your big toe joint starts in the arch of your feet. Hold pressure in this area as you move your finger (or you have them move their finger) in a circular motion.
- Push a thumb into the center of the bottom of the foot, beneath the toes and where the arch begins. Hold the pressure there and move in a circular motion.
- Lift up the toes of the foot as your other hand uses its thumb to push into the center of the heel. Hold this position for a minute.

# Aromatherapy

If you're looking for natural remedies for back and neck pain, there are plenty of treatments to choose from. Aromatherapy is one of the more popular ones, as it's not only effective, but also quite pleasant to incorporate into your life.

In order to create these aromatherapy blends, you will need to find essential oils. These can be ordered through online venues or from health care retailers in your area.

Some easy aromatherapy recipes techniques to use include:

## For When the Pain is Really Bad

4 drops chamomile essential oil
4 drops rosemary essential oil
4 drops ginger essential oil
14 drops lavender essential oil
½ ounce carrier oil - like almond, olive, or sesame

This will help to soothe the muscles and help them to release tension that may be built up. Simply mix these oils together and apply to the skin. If you should find that your skin is irritated in any way, simply add more of your chosen carrier oil to further dilute the essential oils.

## For Moderate Pain

2 drops chamomile essential oil
2 drops birch essential oil
2 drops eucalyptus essential oil
2 drops black pepper essential oil
2 drops lavender essential oil
½ ounce of carrier oil

When put onto the skin when the pain first starts, this concoction can often help to prevent pain from becoming too intolerable.

**How To Win Your War Against Back Pain**

The main concern with most cases of back pain is that you are simply too tense and you need something to calm you down so that your muscles don't tighten.

To deal with tension, try adding some of these essential oils or simply the fragrances to your life. For example, you can add a few drops of the oils to your favorite lotions or dot the diluted oils onto your wrists to smell whenever the pain occurs.

- Lavender oil
- Eucalyptus
- Rosemary
- Clary sage

Choose an essential oil that suits you and makes you feel calmer. Try burning incense or lighting scented candles to further enhance the effects of this therapy.

# <u>Stretching</u>

Of course, if your back and neck pain stem from muscular tension, you will want to make sure you are stretching yourself out as much as possible. To reap the most benefits from this practice, you will need to stretch on a daily basis, preferably several times throughout the day.

- ***Touching your toes*** – Since the hamstrings are generally the tightest part of the body because of our sedentary lifestyles, it's no wonder that they contribute to lower back pain. To help release this tightness, try reaching for your toes as often as you can. Try not to keep the knees straight, but rather try to keep them soft so that you're not hurting yourself in the process.

- ***If you can't touch your toes*** – Place a chair in front of you and lean forward until your arms rest on the chair. This still helps to loosen your back, but prevents you from reaching too far and overstraining yourself. This is a good place to start when you already have back pain.

- ***Side reaches*** – When you are sitting or standing, try to reach your arms up over your head and slightly lean to the side without turning your body. The key is that you shouldn't change your gaze, so keep your head forward. This helps the rest of your body stay forward too.

# Reduce The Stress In Your Life

Many more doctors feel that back and neck pain are actually caused by the stress that you have in your life, rather than injuries or other traumas. So, if you can reduce the stress in your life, you will reduce the incidence of back pain.

Here are some helpful tips to begin to reduce your stress:

- **Create 'me' time**

  Too often, we over-schedule ourselves and never have a free moment to spare for ourselves. This is unhealthy and it can also add to your stress levels. Instead, try to carve out at least ten minutes of 'me' time each day where you're only responsible for yourself and what you want to do.

- **Establish boundaries**

  With cell phones and the internet, it's harder than ever to escape from work. But in order to keep stress at bay, you need to be able to turn off your work life and turn on your relaxation. Create clear boundaries as to when your work day begins and when it ends. Try not to do any work outside of those times and tell others that you will not work outside of those times.

- **Ask for help**

  When we're really stressed, we tend to knuckle down and not ask for help, thinking it makes us look weak to ask. But in the end, this lack of help makes us resentful and possibly even more stressed than we need to be. Ask for help when you need it. People like to help, but only you can tell them when it's necessary.

- **Take time away**

  About 75% of working adults today aren't taking their vacation time from work. Be sure to take this time to get away from the office and unwind. Travel with friends or family and learn how to decompress.

- **Vent your frustrations**

  Instead of bottling up your stress, write down everything that bugs you during the day and then throw away or burn that piece of paper before you go to bed. That will signify that you are done being frustrated and you can relax.

# Lower Right Back Pain Treatment May Indicate Specific Problems

The back pain at the lower part is prevalent in individuals of middle ages, this is because this is the most active period of a person's life. In the middle ages people tend to do a lot of work, get involved in lot of stressful exercises which leads to back pains and other pains as the case may be. One can experience back pain at either the lower right part or at the lower left part as the case might be.

There are two different types of treatments that can be prescribed by the doctor for someone suffering from back pains, he can prescribe a back pain treatment for the lower right or for the lower left. These prescriptions do not just arise once you get to the hospital, the first thing that happens is that, the medical doctor will conduct an examination to really know the gravity and extent of the pain. Most times an X-ray examination is carried out, this will show the doctor the seriousness of the case, elaborating whether or not the internal parts of the body are tampered with, which might be the root cause of the pain.

Once the actual cause of the back pain at the lower right part has been identified, a prescription is given to the patient for the treatment of the pain. There are times when the method of treatment given was not in any way effective in bringing a permanent relief to the patient. Some cases even become more complicated after the treatment process and this should serve as a warning to medical practitioners to only prescribe therapies that have been tested and proved effective to patients suffering from back pains and from any other pains. This is necessary because, it will help to restrict the complications that arise from badly treated back pains.

Care should be taken to always identify the cause of the problem before commencing with the treatment of that problem. This is another way to avoid complicating the issues concerning the back pains at the lower right.

Actually, most pains experienced at the lower right of the back might be a result of a greater problem in the internal part of the body. It could be that the pain is coming from the affected lumbar spine and you are only feeling the resultant effect at the lower right region of the back. You may be experiencing pain as a result from the sciatic, it could also be symptoms of disc

**How To Win Your War Against Back Pain**

herniation. And these pains may be experienced when you either sneeze or cough. The important fact to note is that back pains are usually on the increase whenever the patient is physically active and the pain reduces when the level of activity is reduced, especially when the patient is at rest. Hence, it is advisable to reduce your level of activity if you have a problem with back pains at the lower right part or at any part at all.

If your liver is affected in anyway it may affect the lower right part of the back, causing pains in that region. Pains at the lower right part of the back can also arise from excessive lifting of weights and carrying of heavy objects. Even carrying the back pack at the back fro long can possibly lead to back pains. What ever the cause, get help and treat the pain to experience relief.

# The Truth Behind Electric Waves For Back Pain Relief

The electric wave stimulation is a very good treatment for the relief of back pains. This treatment method is known as the TENS treatment in which electric waves are penetrated into the body through the use of special patches attached on top of the skin. The current flows through the patches into the human body with the aim of bring about a relief to the back pain experienced. This can also be called the electric stimulation method where the body is stimulated hence eradicating the pain felt.

From different researches conducted on the treatment of back pain with the electric wave stimulation method, has been discovered that this method does not have a high percentage record of success. It has not yet been proved to be very successful as a treatment method for chronic or acute pains at the back. But, it will do well as a means of treating normal or mild back pains. Recent records says that the stimulation of electric wave method and placebo has about the same potential since they are both ineffective in the eradication of serious back pains.

Moreover, it has also been discovered that the electric wave stimulation method is very effective in the eradication of labor pains and pregnancy pains. This treatment method can be used to relief the pregnant woman from the pains experienced in pregnancy and also to reduce the effect of labor prior to the delivery of the child.

Basically, before the application of the patches on the skin of the patient, a base cream is applied to help the passage of the electric current through the body from the device. Studies show that this method of treatment originated from ancient times in Greece. But, in those times the equipment used to transfer the current was different from what is obtainable today.

This electric wave stimulation can be used to stimulate sexually, but this method of use is not very popular. the most popular use of the electric wave stimulation is as a treatment method of back pains. It was recorded that Benjamin Franklin certified this method of treatment after he used it for the treatment of his back pain and experienced relief - this increased the popularity of the electric wave stimulation method in the treatment of back pain.

**How To Win Your War Against Back Pain**

There are different types of back pains an the type depends on the severity of the pain, if the pains are very tough and are temporary it is an acute back pain, but if the pains are serious and long lasting then it is a chronic back pain. Some people only experience mild back pains which can not be compared to the seriousness of the acute or chronic pains.

The important thing you should understand if you are having any type of back pain, is that you should make sure the method of treatment is reliable before you use it.

# The Possible Side Effects Of Chiropractic Treatment

There are some side effects associated with the chiropractic therapy, so every one attempting to use that method of treatment should be in the know about the different side effects associated with this kind of treatment method. The basic foundation of the chiropractic practice is the fact that the spine is the control room of the whole body. By this, the chiropractic therapy is a basic necessity if you want the whole body to be perfectly ordered then this therapy should not be avoided in any way.

The spine is the center of concentration for the chiropractice professionals, it is believed that if any one is experiencing pain in any part of the body, it is as a result of the wrong position or the mal functioning of the spine. With this believe system, the spine of individuals are carefully massaged to the proper position so as to eradicate the pain felt at any part of the body. And when this is done, it has been discovered that the pain was really eradicated.

Most medical practitioners do not believe that the chiropractic treatment is purely medical since it does have it roots in medicine. This is why it does not have a wide acceptation around the world by medical practitioners.

When you are experiencing any kind of pain you should carry out a survey of the chiropractic treatment method knowing all you need to know before actually accepting this therapy as a way of reducing or eradicating the pain from your body. Once you have accepted the treatment method the practitioner will then begin to start working on your body, concentrating on the spine to bring about the total wholeness of the body. It will be good to know for sure that the chiropractor can really do the job well before surrendering your self to his or her treatment. If you get to use an unserious person your body will pay dearly for the mistakes.

Another thing you should really know is the side effects associated with this type of treatment, with this you can determine whether to continue or to stop the chiropractic therapy. But, the side effects associated with the chiropractic treatment is very mild, They are just little aches experienced in one path of the body or the other, it can be as small as a minor headache or even a slight pain at different parts of the body as the case may be.

**How To Win Your War Against Back Pain**

Most of the side effects experienced are just minor pains as the result of the massaging of the spine. Definitely, one is to experience pain as a result of the chiropractor working seriously on the spine at the back of the body.

Get information from all those that have used the chiropractic therapy to get rid of all kinds of pains, with this information you can now make an informed decision as at what to do. This investigation will certainly lead you to the right chiropractor that will treat you properly, putting an end to the pains experienced,

# Neck Pain Exercises Can Help

If you are experiencing neck pain, and have visited you medical for examinations, then you need to go ahead to exercise your neck for better and faster results. There are several neck exercises for you to learn and practice, but be careful to avoid mistakes since this can complicate the problem instead. These exercises involve a lot of body movements and is needed to help reduce the pain in the neck, to also prevent the stiffness of the neck. If this is done regularly and consistently for a period of time you will discover that the neck will begin to move easily without much pain.

By doing this regular exercises, you will also discover that your level of activity will be on the increase and the pain will gradually decrease. If you are experiencing chronic pains in your neck that has made it very difficult or you to easily move your neck, the best exercise will be the moderate movement of your neck from left to right - that way you will soon discover that you can now easily move your neck without much stress or pain.

Consistency is the only way out with the exercise method of treating neck pains. This means that you should continue the exercises without stopping until the desired result is seen, in this case, it will be when the neck is completely back to normal and every pain eradicated. When the neck exercises are done several times a day and regularly every day, the path to a pain less neck is created and the patient will soon enjoy relief from the excruciating neck pains. But, you should slowly move your neck and avoid very fast movements so you will not complicate the neck pain.

There are different ways to exercise your neck,  if you are experiencing neck pains. The first one was treated above, and another way will be the stretching of your neck, instead of the side to side movements of the neck. These stretching movements will help you continue the normal free movements as it used to be.

Another way will be the bending neck exercise, all you will need to do in this case is to carefully move your head up and down. The upward and downward movement of the neck will liberate the neck, restoring flexibility to the neck; it also reduces the neck pain.

**How To Win Your War Against Back Pain**

Practice the breathing exercise along with the neck exercises, you will breathe in and out, dragging your breathe. The breathing exercise will help reduce the tension and cause all the muscle around the neck and body to relax, while exercising the neck region as well.

Be sure to check with your doctor before proceeding with these exercises to relieve neck pains.

# Treatment For Chronic Back Pain Is The First Step To Recovery

The most common type of pain experienced by majority is the chronic type of back pain. But in actual sense the factors that bring about this kind of pain differs from one person to another. But, whether the source of pain differ from individual to individual the treatment of this pain in not different, since the same method of treatment is applied to almost all the cases of chronic pains at the back. In most cases, folks tend to offer self treatment when ever there is an issue of back pain, believing that a simple home remedy will do the job, but, when all their efforts fail and the pain continues they run to the hospital for medical attention.

The fact is that one should always go to the hospitals at the first signs of a chronic pain at the back. This is because you do not really know what is responsible for the pain. Without the proper knowledge of the cause of the pain there can not be a lasting remedy, in fact, people end up complicating the issue whenever they try self medication and they end up in more pains than in the beginning. It can become over bearing causing serious distractions since one will not be able to concentrate on the task at hand due to the severe pain experienced.

The use of Ice packs, pain relieving drugs from the drug shop and other means are some of the remedies one may try to use at home for self medication in the treatment of chronic pain at the back. Like I said earlier, the best solution is to consult your doctor, so that a medical examination will be conducted to determine the actual cause, because a problem known is a problem solved. That does not mean that the home remedies are ineffective, they are very effective, because there are times when chronic pains like this are actually treated at home and the pains disappeared after a short while.

A chronic pain is the that kind of pain that has lasted for a while at your back, if the pain you are experiencing does not leave after initial treatments then it must be a chronic pain and it will last for a minimum period of about three months.

It is good for you to visit the doctor for treatment if you are having chronic pains at the back. The very first thing the doctor will do will be to conduct different types of investigations or examination to determine the cause and the extent of the pain. Once the source and the nature

**How To Win Your War Against Back Pain**

of the pain has been identified, treatment will be given by the doctor. Some physical exercises can be recommended to help you with the pain.

There are times when the doctor will just refer you the chiropractor for chiropractic therapy to be used as a means to eradicating the pain. With this therapy the chronic pain at the back of the body will become a thing of the past, never ever occurring again.

# Managing Chronic Pain Including Chronic Neck Pain

Whenever one recovers from either a traumatic situation or surgical operation there is always an acute pain experienced which is usually not permanent but temporary - it might last for some days or weeks depending on the conditions attached to it. In some cases once the problem that brought about the pain is treated the pain will naturally go away. There is another kind of pain experienced known as chronic pain, in this case, it is constant and does not subside easily as in the case of the acute pain; it can actually persist for several years. Chronic neck pain, back pain, headaches, cancer pains, arthritis are different examples of chronic pains experienced by people all around the world.

Before you begin treating a chronic pain, one must first discover the exact part of the body that is causing the pain, once this is discovered the solution is already in view. If the source of a problem is discovered then the problem is solved, since that area becomes the area of concentration in the application of treatment. Whenever a chronic pain is felt on any part of the body, it is always wise to investigate properly to uncover the cause and seek for ways to stop the pain, this can be done through the help of medical practitioners, but, most times even the most experienced doctors find it hard to uncover the direct cause of some pains.

It is not so easy to completely eradicate these chronic pains, although there are many methods of treatment available. In most cases one has to use about two to three methods together to get rid of these pains. A major area of concentration in this case is the issue of chronic pains in the neck, which is experienced around the neck, there are different factors that can contribute to a neck pain with different sources and diverse methods of treatment. Whatever the case is, do not leave a neck pain to continue without treatment or it will become more complicated with the passage of time. The most important thing is to find a way to relieve the pain so as to go on with work as usual, even if the pain is not completely eradicated.

People suffering chronic pains can also help themselves with the kind of food they eat, if your diet plan is not balanced, it will be wise to get a healthy balanced diet plan to reduce the pain. In addition to the above mentioned, you should also exercise properly and get enough rest, sleeping at least five hours a day, that way you will discover that the pain is reduced and your activity level increased.

**How To Win Your War Against Back Pain**

Acupuncture is another way to easily relieve chronic pains, in this case all that is needed is the puncturing of special nerve points with fine needles or even by laser beams, this will bring about a fast relieve from the pains. In all, make sure you visit your doctor to examine you and offer the best possible treatment to cure the chronic pain or neck pain.

# The Art Of Getting Insurance Coverage For Chiropractic Care

It has been a difficult task in the past to get an insurance company offering a cover for the chiropractic treatment of back pains. This is as a result of the fact that this method of treatment is not accepted as a purely medical practice by other medical practitioners. And because of this most insurance companies do not offer cover this, even though the chiropractic treatment is very cheap and affordable than other form of treatment, since it does not involve any from of surgery as the others do.

But, with the passage of time, the chiropractic treatment is become more popular as a result of the successes recorded by this method of treatment, it has become a valuable method of treating back pains. Due to this improvement many insurance companies are offering cover for this method of treatment. In recent times it can become very easy for you to get a cover for the chiropractic treatment included in your health insurance, but most time you have to actually convince some of these companies to do this for you, which might be very difficult and time consuming at times.

For instance, it can become very difficult to get the insurance firm to pay for the chiropractic treatment even if it was recommended by the physician at the primary health care.

The insurance care policies that cover the chiropractic treatment are the alternative and complementary policies. The payments and coverages given by the insurance companies that offer the chiropractic treatment cover are the same with all other insurance coverage policies. Get the insurance company that will provide a coverage for this method of treatment with a favorable payment plan and discount plan.

The difficulty involved in getting the right insurance coverage for your health plan is always a hideous task. In fact you can never actually get the insurance plan that favors you completely meeting all your needs. If you finally get one it will seem as if you just hit a jackpot, because frankly speaking it is very rare to see such. Where will you find an insurance cover that completely takes care of all your medical bills - you can hardly find that. And then getting one that will agree to cover for a treatment method that is not considered as a purely medical treatment will be like pouring water into a basket. Because it might just be an effort in futility.

**How To Win Your War Against Back Pain**

The best thing to always do before signing up an insurance policy will be to do an in-depth research of all the policies covered by the insurance company, knowing all the necessary details before going ahead to sign up for that health insurance. This will help you to know if the insurance company offers a cover for the chiropractic treatment of back pains or any other pain.

# Know All The Causes And Treatment Of Lower Back Pain

Lower back pain is the most popular type of back pain, eight out of every ten people suffering back pain is a lower back pain. This excruciating pain originates from several sources too numerous to mention and it can affect anybody without age restrictions, it has been discovered though, that people between the ages of thirty to fifty are more prone to experiencing lower back pain.

The habit of hanging back packs at the back by most young people is another cause of pain at the back. The fact that you do not involve in much work that lead to pain at the lower back and when you do too much work you may also develop pain in the lower part of the back. The origin of pains at the lower back can differ from Peron to person. But, if you are experiencing a lower back pain it will be good to know the source of the pain so as to deal with it promptly.

The age of an individual, a disc that is ruptured, spinal degeneration, sciatica, heavy lifting etc. are one of the major sources of pains at the lower part of back. The important thing to note is that once any of these bring about a back pain, do not hesitate to treat the condition promptly to avoid complications. Do a search, investigate thoroughly to know the major sources of back pains and then you will be able to get a hold of the situation. This should be done whenever symptoms of back pain arises.

It is always important for people to develop and maintain the proper posture and ways of standing, sitting and movement, this helps to prevent back pains especially the lower back pains. It has been observed that those that do not stand, sit and move properly tend to be prone to body pains, mostly back pains. Different employers have spent a lot of money sensitizing their employees on the need for good postures and all it takes to leave free from back pains. And, this is very necessary since prevention is always better than cure.

There are many ways to treat pains at the lower back, and the best treatment is based upon the gravity of the pain experienced. If the issue is very complicated then the patient will be taken in for surgery. However, most lower back pains do not end up in surgery. There is a simple way of handling pains from injuries that works perfectly: Once there is an injury or accident, quickly apply some ice on the injured part, and continue this regularly for about two days. With this you

**How To Win Your War Against Back Pain**

will discover that the pain is reduced and that there is no swelling experienced. This system helps to avoid the complications attached to any accident or injury that may affect the lower back or any part of the body.

Basically, the medical treatment of pains at the lower back involves the ingestion of anti-inflammatory and reliever of pain medication for about three days. After this further actions will be taken if the first phase of treatment did not eradicate the pain. If the first phase did not help remove or reduce the pain, examinations will be conducted to probe into the cause and extent of the back pain. For instance an x-ray examination will be taken to actually see the condition of the back as to determine the nature of the pain. After all treatments, it will be best to practice some exercises to heal and repair the damages affecting the back.

# Chiropractic Treatment Of Back Pain Doesn't Have To Be A Last Resort

Chiropractic therapy for relieving back pain is a method of treating back pain where the back is massaged and the vertebra put back in the right place. People use this method as a last option when treating back pains, it must have been that all other options failed and the chiropractic remained as the last option.

I believe this method has not enjoyed the patronage of medical professionals, maybe because they do not understand the source of treatment as being medical. This accounts for the reason why most doctors offer this treatment as a last option when all the methods they used did not produce the desired result.

For example, if a patient comes with a problem of back pains, the doctor may first offer something to relieve the pain, when the pain continues of some days, an x-ray examination is carried out to determine the nature and extent of the pain. After thorough analysis, other complex medications are offered even with physical therapy. When all the doctors attempts prove futile in the eradication of pains at the back, the chiropractic therapy is suggested to the patient as a last option.

It really does not have to be this way, since the chiropractic method of treating back pains is very potent. It has help a lot of people get rid of all types of back pains, and should be used by many as a first option in the treatment of back pains. Just think about it, will it not be better to use the most effective method first and be relieved immediately, than trying many ineffective methods. This will only waste your time and cause you to remain in an agonizing pain for a long time when a better way exist to rid your back of that pain.

The chiropractic treatment is an easy one and does not involve much, it is just an adjustment of the back, putting it back to the normal position which will erase the pain, leaving a relaxed feeling on your nerves. The practitioner only need to use his or her arm on your back fixing the vertebrae with short but quick movements, some times the use of ice is implored to relax the nerves of the patient if there are some feelings of pains noticed during the course of treatment.

**How To Win Your War Against Back Pain**

If that is the case, a break is given to the patient to relax and he or she is stimulated electrically prior to the next session of the chiropractic therapy.

Another obvious fact about the chiropractic therapy, is the fact that it is not a permanent treatment, since one can come back again and again for back adjustments whenever the pain is felt at the back. This goes to show that the back adjustments does not provide a lasting or permanent treatment to the problem of back pain.

# Sports Medicine Physician Salaries - An Analysis

The physicians of sports medicine are just the medical practitioners that have an in-depth knowledge of the different types of drugs available for the treatment of those involved in sports. These doctors specialize in the various sport medicines and the various ways to administer them to patients.

Physicians of sport medicine are there with the sole goal to improve the performance of those involve in the different sport. These medications also help these sport men and women to reduce their level of inability and injuries to the lowest minimal. This can either be at the workplace, at sports and also the school.

## Those that Specialize in Sports Medicine

The specialist involved in sport medicine spends a lot of time in training because of the delicate and demanding nature of the job. They also have to do a lot of studies and research in conjunction with a good qualification before setting out to practice this profession. Salaries given to these specialist of sport medicine differ a lot, the amount of money given to one will be different from the other since the level of qualification is different because that is the measuring standards used in determining the wages of these special health workers.

Specialists in sports medicine have their focus in the application of the medical skills and knowledge on those involved in sports. This helps to bring about high level of productivity and effectiveness within the sporting communities. They are there to help all those involved in sports perform very well with the perfect working body system. A sport man or woman can actually achieve greats things with a strong, healthy body system. That is why the function of the sports medical specialists can not be under estimated.

The knowledge of science and medicine is applied into exercise and sports, this is the actual summary of what the specialists in sports medicine are involved in. They possess an in-depth knowledge and application in the treatment of all types of sport related injuries. These specialists are needed whenever a sporting event is taking place, or when one is even exercising in the gym, where ever there is a sporting event - they must be there because they are to handle and treat all injuries derived from the various sporting activities.

## The Factors that Determine their Salaries

Two hundred and forty dollars and four hundred and seventy five dollars are the two different categories of the payment schedule for the specialist of sport medicines. This result is the recent result of the Medical association in the United States.

Many factors are used to consider the amount of salary any specialist of the sport medicine will receive. These factors are the age of the specialist and the level of experienced acquired - this will determine the amount of money the specialist will receive. The sex of the specialist can also influence the amount of the salary the specialist will receive. The more patients the specialists attends to the more money he or she makes.

# Going Through Sciatica Therapy For Your Pain

There are many therapies existing now for the treatment of the sciatica pain. Medical professionals mostly recommend that their clients go through these therapies are a way to relief the pain: the prescription of pain relieving drugs comes as a last resort after the therapy.

Many medical practitioners in recent times are now with the habit of requiring their patients to undergo the therapy of sciatica so as to certify the real existence of the pain before proceeding with the normal medication. The importance of this therapy is to build the patients mind set so that the pain will be controlled.

This special therapy for sciatica is also known as the therapy for cognitive behavior. This is a psychological therapy which concentrates on the mind of the patient, working on the mindset. It tries hard to change the feelings, emotions and the behavior of the patient - hence reducing or completely eradicating the pain felt. In this case, the patient is made to live with the pain without actually feeling the pain because of the change of the process of his or her thinking pattern. By this the patient eventually conquers the pain.

No matter how hard the medical practitioners or the psychologist try, some patients cases are exceptions, since the therapy does not work at all with them, no matter how hard it is used, it might only be useful for other things for such people. This therapy helps to build up the patients in many different ways. For instance, if a patient goes for this therapy, he or she will learn how to endure pains, in other words this person develops the high tolerance of pain, which would have not be possible without the therapy.

Apart from the ability to endure pains the patient is able conquer all forms of depression and also have to eventually improve on his relationship with people and every other aspect of the patient 's life will experience an improvement as a result of this therapy. This makes this therapy very important and it is loved by all that participate in it.

It really sounds funny to think about the fact that someone's mind will be worked upon to make him or her believe that there is no pain experienced when the pain is still there, some times individuals find it hard to accept this. And, some patients do not like the idea of sitting in midst of

**How To Win Your War Against Back Pain**

many people going through the therapy of sciatica in the midst of a crowd. But some love being in the midst of the crowd enjoying the group therapy, because there are a lot of things to be learnt from both the therapist and from others in the discussion of different kinds of topics that are relevant to the case.

It has become mandatory for every one suffering from the sciatica pain to undergo the therapy for sciatica.

# Different Kinds Of Upper Right Back Pain Treatment Can All Help

Any type of pain one experiences has the ability to incapacitate the sufferer of the pain, regardless of the type of pain or the region of the body affected. The effect of back pains on the body can be very devastating, since one is no longer able to concentrate on the task at hand due to the distraction created by the excruciating pain on the body - it is very difficult to take one's mind off that. But, the good news I have for you is that no matter the type or gravity of pain experienced there is always a solution that will completely eradicate the pain, leaving you happy and very relieved to concentrate on other important issues.

Now, the back pain at the upper right is not a very common type, since the majority of people suffering from back pains usually complain of experiencing pain at the lower back - this is the well known  kind of back pain experienced. The back pain at the upper right is a special kind and there are many ways to solve this problem. The major function of the upper part of the back is to hold up the upper part of the body as a support system for all the part of the body there. For instance, the upper back region is responsible for holding up the neck and the head in position. From this, the importance of this upper back section becomes very obvious, making it very necessary for us to always address any problems related to this section of the body.

Pains at the upper right part of the back mainly arise as a result of the wrong use of the back or as a result of the wrong body posture, the latter is almost always the case since most people are of the habit of not sitting or standing properly - hence developing back pains at this region of the back. Most times when the muscles are irritated or are not functioning properly the result is a back pain at the upper right section. The factors that contribute to this type of pain can not be exhausted here, so only the main factors are stated above.

If you discover that you are experiencing pain at the upper right region of your back, the first thing to do will be to visit your doctor. At the hospital a series of examination will be conducted to ascertain the real cause of the pain. One of the most important examination will be an x-ray to view the internal part of the body, this will show the source and the gravity of the back pain. This is very necessary so as to know exactly what the problem is.

**How To Win Your War Against Back Pain**

The most effective treatment method for back pains at the upper right part, is the chiropractic therapy, in this method the spine is treated to bring about relief to the pain. You can also use acupuncture to effectively remove the pain felt at the upper right region of the back, in every method of treatment applied, drugs will be given to you by the doctor to relief the pains.

# Scoliosis Surgery - Upper Back Pain Is Not Due To Scoliosis Surgery

There is no link between pain in the region of the upper back and scoliosis surgery always. Those who suffer with scoliosis may not always require surgery nor is back pain a symptom of this problem always. This is a condition where the spine has an unnatural curvature which is over ten degrees and is a congenital condition that is present at the time of birth and is caused by vertebral anomalies. There are sub classifications of scoliosis which occur at different stages in life like infantile, juvenile, adolescent and adult scoliosis. This is also a secondary symptom of cerebral palsy or muscular atrophy.

**Some common symptoms of scoliosis**

Some of the symptoms of scoliosis which are quite common are one side of the rib cage could appear higher than the other, the tilting of the body to one side, shoulders are at uneven height, one leg may be longer than the other, or in women the asymmetric size or location of the breast. Sometimes surgery is required for this problem or for the pain, however, pain is not always associated with or a typical symptom of scoliosis. In case a child or young person who has scoliosis also has sever back pain, the doctor who is taking care of him or her would have to conduct some tests to see if there is some other underlying problem too. Lower back pain in youngsters may not be a symptom associated with scoliosis, but if untreated and if it appears in adults it could be due to scoliosis. So an adult with a similar problem to a child may require surgery to relieve the pain.

**The reasons for conducting scoliosis surgery**

Normally doctors prefer not to indulge in surgery for adolescents or children who suffer from scoliosis. However, if the problem is causing them problems with breathing, incessant pain, or if they appear cosmetically gross, then the doctors would resort to scoliosis surgery. Surgery is also required for patients who have spina bifida or cerebral palsy.

The scoliosis surgery that is done most often for upper back pain, is with instrumentation for spinal fusion. For this surgery, a bone from a donor is harvested in the patients body in some other part and then grafted to the vertebrae. With this the vertebral column turns rigid and forms one solid mass of bone. Thus preventing the scoliosis to become worse and prevents the curvature from increasing.

# Tendinitis And Other Causes Of Neck, Left Shoulder And Upper Back Pain

Upper back pain, left shoulder pain and neck pain are a condition that is common to most Americans and they suffer from this sort of pain from time to time in their life. This pain is sometimes not too severe but could also be unbearable and beyond tolerance sometimes. Reasons for pain in the upper back, left shoulder and neck is often a problem with the shoulder joint. The shoulder joint is very susceptible to injuries like sprains, strains and tears. Because of this injury there can be inflammation of the joints, muscles, ligaments and of the bursa, causing immense discomfort and pain. A shoulder injury can give rise to pain in the upper back, left shoulder and neck region also. The motion of the arm is allowed by the muscles, joints and tendons of the shoulders and any injury to this portion of the body will result in immediate discomfort and difficulty in movement.

**Causes of tendinitis**

Tendinitis is a the connecting link of the muscles, tissues and bones which is a cord. Inflammation of this cord caused by too much usage of the muscles and any injury that might have occurred results in this kind of pain in the neck and shoulder regions. Upper back pain, pain in the left shoulder and the neck are caused by rotator cuff injuries. The area for the rotator cuff is very small and any inflammation with swelling can be the cause of a lot of discomfort and pain and also the arm that is affected will be weakened.

**A change in lifestyle is a preventive measure**

Sometimes a change in one's life style can prevent this sort of a problem with back pain and pain in the neck and shoulder. Of course, accidents cannot be prevented but you could try and lead a healthier life to avoid degenerative diseases and weakening of the muscles. Keeping fit and exercising regularly is one way to strengthen your muscles and avoiding these sort of discomforts and protecting your back and neck and shoulders. You should ensure that you are careful when lifting weights, keep a good posture and do not let stress cause you these sort of problems. In case there is some physical activity that you have to do that causes you discomfort, try and change the way you do it so that it does not cause you unwanted pain.

**How To Win Your War Against Back Pain**

## See a doctor if pain persists

For a persisting pain it is always better to seek medical advice. The doctor will probably do some diagnostic clinical tests and x-rays and scans to evaluate what the problem is. Once he is sure of what is causing the discomfort in the neck, back and shoulders, treatment will be provided. It may be a neurological problem or something to do with the muscles and ligaments.

# Causes Of Neck Pain And Headaches

Athletes and sports people often have headaches and neck pains which originate at the nape of the neck and move to their heads via the temples, eyes and the neck. Describing this accurately to the doctor is important because then the doctor will know whether it is a referred pain due to an injury in some other part of the body. The headaches are of different kinds and of different levels of severity and what most people do not realize that there is a link between the headache and the neck pain. Stiffness and pain in the neck can cause pain whenever the person tries to move the head. Often this stiffness is associated with headaches too. Stiffness in the neck is often accompanied by headaches.

## Sleeping in a wrong position and neck pain

A stiff neck or what is in medical terms referred to as a cervical spasm is not a serious disorder but is one that causes a lot of discomfort. This is something that usually comes about with sleeping in a wrong posture or using a pillow that does not support the head and neck properly. This brings about muscular pain and the result is a head ache and a neck pain.

Poor posture causes head ache and neck pain and the person does not even realize that he has a bad posture and continues to do it until the pain starts and keeps getting worse. Some of the bad postures that cause head aches and pain in the neck are walking with a slouch, carrying a weighty bag on your shoulder, reading while lying in bed, the computer being too high or low while working on it for long hours, and sitting in a twisted curled position in front of the television.

## Medical reasons for headache and neck pains

There are also medical conditions that cause headaches and neck pains and not just bad posture that does this. Meningitis and high blood pressure are also causes for this kind of discomfort and pain. A bad neck pain which gets worse when the chin is moved downwards is a symptom of meningitis. After an accident if there is concussion there is neck pain and headache also.

**How To Win Your War Against Back Pain**

In case any person is suffering from constant neck pains and headaches they should always get a medical opinion for this and ascertain the reason for this. This sort of a symptom should not be neglected if it persists for some time and proper medical treatment should be started for the cause as soon as possible. If there is nausea along with he pain and a tingling feeling in the arms the doctor should be consulted immediately. The doctor may suggest some simple home exercises to relieve you of this discomfort too.

# Diagnosing Lower Back Pain

Back pain will inhibit millions of Americans this year, and for some, the pain can be excruciating. Back pain can be caused by a large number of injuries or conditions, thus making a proper diagnosis both difficult and critical. Back pain that occurs with other symptoms like fever and chills, severe abdominal pain or bladder and bowel problems can be an indication of a serious medical condition, and should be evaluated by your doctor immediately.

Lower back pain is classified into one of three categories, based on a description of how the pain is distributed throughout the body. These three categories are axial lower back pain (also known as mechanical or simple back pain), radicular lower back pain (also known as sciatica) and lower back pain with referred pain. We will now briefly examine the most common causes and treatments for each of these categories.

The most common type of lower back pain is axial. This pain is confined to the lower back area and does not radiate into the surrounding portions of the body. There are many causes of axial lower back pain, such as a degenerated disc or damage to the muscles, ligaments or tendons. However, in most cases, the treatment of axial lower back pain is not dependant on the cause.

The usual treatment is rest, exercises or physical therapy, the use of hot and/or cold compresses and various common pain medications. The exceptions to this would be for chronic pain or pain that is so severe that it wakes you up at night. In these cases, one should see their doctor.

Radicular lower back pain is caused by compression of the lower spinal nerve, leading to pain that radiates down the thighs and legs. The most common nerve affected is the sciatic nerve, which runs down the back of the thigh and calf into the food. Sciatica may cause greater pain in the leg than in the back. This nerve compression can be caused by a herniated disc, a narrowing of the passage through which the nerve travels the spine, diabetes or nerve root injuries.

Usually sciatica is treated with physical therapy and medication for a period of six to eight weeks. If the pain persists, surgery may be done to relieve the compression.

**How To Win Your War Against Back Pain**

Lower back pain with referred pain which spreads to other areas of the body can be caused by the same conditions which cause axial lower back pain, and the treatment is similar. It needs to be carefully differentiated from radicular lower back pain, in which the pain spreads in very specific paths along certain nerves.

Most instances of back pain can be treated successfully with a combination of rest, physical therapy, hot and cold packs and pain medication. Only with severe or persistent pain should a more drastic treatment, such as surgery, be considered.

# Chiropractors And Back Pain

Chiropractors treat health problems that are associated with the body's muscular, nervous, and skeletal systems, especially the spine. The science of chiropractic is mainly based around spinal manipulation.  With manipulation, a practitioner will use their hands to mobilize, adjust, massage, or stimulate the spine or surrounding tissues.  The purpose of spinal manipulation is to restore joint mobility by applying a controlled force into joints that have become restricted in their movement.

The word chiropractic comes from the Greek words chiro and practices, and roughly means done by hand.

This refers to how a chiropractor will use their hands to manipulate the spine. Chiropractic is a healing discipline based on science. Although its main focus is the relationship between the skeleton and the nervous system, chiropractic is concerned with the entire body.

Chiropractic is by far the most popular form of alternative health care, and uses a holistic approach in its treatment.

Chiropractors believe the correct alignment of the spine is necessary for the nervous system to function properly.

The theory is that the body cannot function and heal itself without the nervous system being free of interference. The interference with these systems impairs the body's normal functions and lowers its resistance to disease. The spine is the most common site of nervous interference because nerves travel from the spinal cord through openings on either side of the spine to get to all of your cells and organs.

Chiropractic adjustments involve applying a controlled, sudden force to a joint. It is a non-invasive, manual procedure that utilizes the skills developed through intensive chiropractic education. Adjustment is a carefully controlled procedure delivered by a skilled practitioner. The primary goal is to decrease pain and to improve range of motion in the joints and supporting tissues.

**How To Win Your War Against Back Pain**

Like other health practitioners, chiropractors will take the patient's medical history, conduct various examinations; and may order laboratory tests in order to make a diagnosis and develop a treatment. X-rays and other diagnostic images are important tools to a chiropractor as they show the position of the spine and its alignment.

Chiropractors practice a drug-free, manual approach to health care that includes patient assessment, diagnosis and treatment. Chiropractors are also trained to recommend therapeutic exercise, to utilize other non-invasive therapies, as well as to provide nutritional, dietary and lifestyle counseling.

Some chiropractors use treatments in addition to spinal manipulation. These include therapy using water, light, massage, ultrasound, electric impulses, acupuncture and heat. They also may apply supports such as straps, tapes, and braces. Chiropractors counsel patients about wellness concepts such as nutrition, exercise, changes in lifestyle, and stress management, but do not prescribe drugs or perform surgery.

Chiropractic training is a 4-year academic program. It consists of both classroom and clinical instruction.

Students are only eligible for chiropractic training after first completing at least three years of college. Students who graduate receive the degree of Doctor of Chiropractic (D.C.). All chiropractors are regulated by their state's license board.

# How To Prevent Back Pain

Simple lower back pain can be caused by straining the muscles, tendon or ligaments of the lower back. Often this is a result of heavy or awkward activity, especially if you are unused to it. Here are some tips to help prevent you from injuring your back, and becoming one of the millions of Americans who suffer from lower back pain.

The most effective prevention is to take care as to how you lift heavy objects. Do not try to lift any significant weight by bending over the object. You should bend your knees and then lift with your legs. Try to keep your back straight and hold the object close to your body. It is important to avoid twisting your body while lifting, which is the most common cause of a slipped disk.

When moving heavy objects, pushing is less stressful than pulling.

Routine activities, such as housework or gardening, can cause back pain. Try to avoid standing flat-footed while bent over. Placing one foot on a small stool or book while washing dishes or ironing can reduce the strain on your back. When vacuuming, try to move your whole body, using your legs to push.

A sedentary lifestyle will contribute to back problems.

Regular exercise will have great benefit to you. You should consider a set of stretching and other exercises to improve the flexibility and strength of the muscles which support your lower back. These include the abdominal muscles, as well as those in the legs and back. Simple exercises like partial sit-ups and bridges can help prevent back pain throughout your life. Obesity is a common cause of back pain. Aerobic exercise can help manage weight concerns. Swimming, jogging or even walking are all activities that will help you lose weight and feel better. Before starting any vigorous activity, make sure you do a proper warm-up with stretching.

In addition to exercise, a proper diet is essential in managing your weight. However, there are also two nutrients, calcium and vitamin D, that help build healthy and strong bones and prevent osteoporosis, which can cause bone fractures that lead to back pain.

**How To Win Your War Against Back Pain**

Many people whose jobs involve sitting for long periods of time experience back pain. It is important to get up and move around regularly. If driving for long periods of time, take the time to stop and get out of your vehicle.

Stretching your muscles and improving blood flow to your lower body will help prevent back pain, as well as help keep you alert for the rest of your trip.

Changing the position in which you sleep can also help prevent back pain. The best positions are either to sleep lying on your side with your legs bent, or lying on your back with a pillow under your knees. A firm mattress is usually the best bet. A sheet of plywood can be placed between the box spring and the mattress in order to increase the firmness of your bed.

# Living With Back Pain

Back pain may be relieved with a variety of techniques.

For most common occurrences of back pain, a regiment of rest, hot and cold compresses, exercise and therapy, as well as various pain medications can be used to reduce the pain and provide a level of comfort.

Rest will be necessary for your back to heal when suffering from acute back pain. However, you should try to maintain as much activity as is comfortable. Getting up and moving around can help ease stiffness and relieve pain.

Hot and cold compresses, used separately or by alternating, can have great benefit in reducing back pain. Heat is used to relax the muscles. It works by dilating the blood vessels, which improves the flow of oxygen to the affected area and reduces pain and muscle spasms. It is important to take care when applying heat to the lower back region. Constant heat for prolonged periods can have a negative effect on the organs in your abdominal region. Do not sleep with a heating pad on your back. Instead, apply heat for no more than 20 to 30 minutes. Cold packs are used to reduce inflammation, such as that from arthritis or injury.

This works by decreasing the size of blood vessels and the flow of blood to the area. Like heat packs, it is important to avoid prolonged application of cold packs.

A simple solution for a cold pack is to take a bag of ice or frozen peas and wrap it in a towel.

Various stretching exercises can be used to reduce back pain by reducing back stiffness and possibly relieving compression on the spine. As well, suitable exercises will strengthen the muscles of the abdomen, buttocks, back and legs, which will provide better support to your back and help relieve pain. Your doctor or physical therapist can show you a set of exercises suitable for your condition. Massage therapy is used by many to relieve back pain. Massage tries to stimulate blood flow to the affected area, and to relax the muscles of the lower back. Registered massage therapists can be found on-line or in your phone book.

**How To Win Your War Against Back Pain**

Nonprescription medicines can be used to reduce pain.

They include analgesic medications like aspirin and acetaminophen (Tylenol), which are meant for general pain relief. Topical analgesics include such as Zostrix, Icy Hot and Ben Gay can be effective in some cases where a pill-based medicine is not. Other medicines, such as NSAIDs, or non-steroidal anti-inflammatory drugs, are used to reduce swelling. These include such nonprescription medications as ibuprofen (Motrin, Advil), ketoprofen (Actron, Orudis) and naproxen sodium (Aleve). Prescription medications are available if these medications do not prove effective.

You should call your family doctor if your pain remains after a couple of weeks, or if you feel any of these other symptoms:

- Pain in your leg below the knee
- Numbness in the legs or groin
- Fever, nausea or vomiting, stomach pain, weakness or sweating
- Loss of control over bathroom functions

# Risk Factors For Back Pain

It is estimated that 80% of all Americans will experience back pain in their lives. This means that it is likely you will suffer from back pain eventually. There are several risk factors that can contribute to the frequency and intensity back pain episodes. By being aware of them, you can modify your behavior to reduce your risk of suffering from back pain.

The most common age to first experience back pain is between 30 and 40. At this time the body is beginning to lose its flexibility. Back pain becomes more common with age, as the number of conditions that can cause back pain increase. Musculoskeletal strains are more common with younger people, while arthritis and degenerative disc disease tend to be leading causes of back pain among seniors.

People who live sedentary lifestyles are more likely to experience back pain than those who engage in regular activity. Those with a higher level of physical fitness generally have stronger muscles in the back, legs and abdomen, all of which help support the back. The exception to this is the so-called "Weekend Warriors", people who engage in vigorous activity only periodically, with little exercise in between. They are at the greatest risk of injuring themselves during their periods of exertion. Those who are least likely to suffer from back pain are those who engage in a moderate level of activity on a regular basis.

Perhaps the most significant risk factor is obesity. The strain of carrying excess weight can contribute greatly to back pain. Regular exercise and a balanced diet can help control obesity, and reduce the frequency of back pain episodes.

Having a job that requires heavy lifting, particularly while twisting or vibrating the spine, can lead to injury and back pain. It is important that if your job involves heavy lifting, pushing or pulling, you should make the effort to use proper techniques in order to protect your back.

Bend your knees and lift with your legs, keeping your back straight. Before starting your day, consider doing a series of stretching and strengthening exercises to loosen your back muscles and help prepare them for the work ahead.

**How To Win Your War Against Back Pain**

A desk job may also lead to back pain, particularly if you sit all day in an uncomfortable chair or have bad posture.  Try to sit straight with your feet firmly planted on the ground.  Make sure your computer monitor is at the correct height, which is usually recommended to be that the top on the monitor is two inches above your eye level. Stretching activities done throughout the day can help to keep your back loose.

Although smoking may not directly cause back pain, it increases your risk of developing low back pain sciatica. Smoking may lead to pain by blocking your body's ability to deliver nutrients to the discs of the lower back.

# Exercising And Back Pain

Exercising is of great benefit both to someone suffering from back pain and for anyone hoping to avoid it in the future. If you are suffering from acute back pain, exercising may not be possible or even a good idea.

However, for chronic back pain, a regular exercise program will probably be recommended by your doctor. Either your physician or a physical therapist can help you in developing an exercise plan that is suitable for you and your condition. You will want to include the following types of exercises.

Stretching exercises are designed to improve the extension of the muscles and soft tissues. This can reduce stiffness and increase range of motion. Typical stretching exercises for the back include lying on your back and raising each leg to your chest, as well as bridges and hamstring stretches.

The purposes of flexion exercises, which are exercises in which you bend forward, are to widen the spaces between the vertebrae. This relieves pressure on the nerves, and stretches the muscles of the back and hips.

They will also strengthen the muscles that support the spine, those of the back, abdomen and legs

With extension exercises, you bend backward. They open up the spinal canal in places and develop muscles that support the spine. Extension exercises may minimize radicular pain, which is pain that radiates to other parts of the body besides the back, especially the legs and lower extremities. Extension exercises include leg lifts and trunk raises.

Aerobic exercise is the type that gets your heart rate elevated for a period of time. It is also known as cardiovascular exercise. It is recommended to get at least 30 minutes of aerobic exercise three times a week. Aerobic exercises are good for working the large muscles of the back and core. For those with back problems, walking, jogging and swimming may be suitable aerobic activities. For back problems, you should avoid exercise that requires twisting or

**How To Win Your War Against Back Pain**

vigorous bending, like aerobics and rowing, as well as contact sports like football or hockey, because these activities may cause more damage to your back. Especially avoid high-impact activities if you have any sort of disc disease. If back pain or your fitness level makes it impossible to exercise 30 minutes at a time, try three 10-minute sessions to start with and work up to your goal.

Obesity is a common cause of back pain. The strain of carrying excess weight can contribute greatly to back pain. Regular exercise and a balanced diet can help control obesity, and reduce the frequency of back pain episodes. Aerobic exercise can help manage weight concerns. Swimming, jogging or even walking are all activities that will help you lose weight and feel better.

If you suffer from back pain, it is important to make sure that you are doing the right exercises and that you are doing them properly. A physical therapist can help you develop proper techniques so that you can derive the maximum benefit for your exercise and avoid injuring yourself further.

# Alternative Therapy For Back Pain

There are a wide variety of alternative treatments for back pain. Most of the studies of these therapies have proved inconclusive. Some people will claim certain treatments will cure anything, especially if they have a financial interest in it. However, many people have obtained benefits from the treatments described below.

Traction involves using pulleys and weights to stretch the back. The rationale behind traction is to pull the vertebrae apart to allow a bulging disc to slip back into place. Some people experience pain relief while in traction, but that relief is usually temporary. Once traction is released back pain is likely to return. Corsets and braces limit the motion of the lumbar spine, provide abdominal support, and correct posture. They are of most use after certain surgeries.

Various injections can be used to relieve chronic back pain if medication and other non-surgical treatments fail. Some of the most commonly used injections include nerve root blocks, facet joint injections, and trigger point injections. Prolotherapy is a treatment in which a sugar solution or other irritating substance is injected into the periosteum, the fibrous tissue covering the bones, in order to strengthen the attachment of tendons and ligaments.

Spinal manipulation is done by chiropractors and osteopathic doctors. With manipulation, a practitioner will use their hands to mobilize, adjust, massage, or stimulate the spine or surrounding tissues. The purpose of spinal manipulation is to restore joint mobility by applying a controlled force into joints that have become restricted in their movement.  Spinal manipulation is not an appropriate treatment for osteoporosis, spinal cord compression, or arthritis.

Transcutaneous Electrical Nerve Stimulation (TENS) uses mild electric impulses to stimulate the nervous system in the pained area. It is thought that TENS may elevate the levels of endorphins, the body's natural pain-numbing chemicals, in the spinal fluid.

Acupuncture is an ancient Chinese practice that is based on the theory that a life force called Qi flows through the body. If the flow is impeded, the body can become ill. Acupuncture involves the insertion of thin needles at precise locations to unblock the flow of Qi, relieving pain and restoring health. Some studies have indicated that inserting and then stimulating needles (by twisting or passing a low-voltage electrical current through them) may foster the production of endorphins.

Acupressure is similar to acupuncture in that it seeks to unblock the flow of Qi.

The difference between acupuncture and acupressure is that no needles are used in acupressure.

Acupressure is more like massage therapy, where a therapist will use their hands, elbows, feet and knees to apply pressure to certain precise portions of the patient's body.

Another type of massage, Rolfing, uses strong pressure on deep tissues in the back to relieve tightness of the fascia, a sheath of tissue that covers the muscles. It seeks to improve posture and structure by manipulating the body's myofascial system

# Surgery For Back Pain

While the majority of treatment for lower back pain is non-surgical, there are some conditions for which surgery is appropriate. As well, in some rare cases, surgery can be used to treat chronic back pain for which other treatments have failed. Below we list some common conditions that may be treated surgically, and describe the treatments used.

A herniated disc occurs when the hard outer coating of the discs, the circular pieces of connective tissue that cushion the vertebrae, are damaged. These discs may leak, irritating nearby nerves. A herniated disc is also known as a ruptured disc. A herniated disk can cause severe sciatica, nerve pain that radiates down the leg.

Herniated discs may be treated surgically by discectomy, either laminectomy, microdiscectomy or laser discectomy. In a laminectomy, part of the lamina, a portion of the bone on the back of the vertebrae, is removed. The herniated disc is then removed through this cut. In microdiscectomy a much smaller incision is made and the doctor uses a magnifying lens to locate the disc. The smaller incision may reduce pain and the disruption of tissues, and it reduces the size of the surgical scar. With a laser discectomy, a laser is used to vaporize the tissue in the disc, reducing its size and relieving pressure on the nerves.

Spinal stenosis is a condition where the spinal canal narrows, compressing the nerves inside. It is often caused by bone spurs which are a result of osteoarthritis. Compression of the nerves can lead to pain, numbness in the legs and the loss of bladder or bowel control. A laminectomy may be used to open up the spinal column remove the lamina and any bone spurs. The procedure is major surgery that requires a short hospital stay and physical therapy afterwards.

Spondylolisthesis is a condition where a vertebra of the slips out of place. As the spine tries to stabilize itself, the joints between the slipped vertebra and adjacent vertebrae can become enlarged. This can pinch nerves, causing low back pain and severe sciatica leg pain. A spinal fusion may be used with a laminectomy.

In spinal fusion, two or more vertebrae are joined together using bone grafts, screws, and rods to prevent slippage of the slipped vertebrae. The bone used for the bone graft usually comes from the hip or pelvis of the patient, although a donor bone may be used. The fused area of the spine becomes immobilized.

Vertebral fractures can be caused by trauma or by osteoporosis. A vertebroplasty injects a cement-like mixture called polymethyacrylate into the fractured vertebra to stabilize the spine. Kyphoplasty inserts a balloon device to help restore the height and shape of the spine before injecting polymethyacrylate to repair the fractured vertebra.

Degenerative disc disease is an aging process where the discs between the vertebrae break down over time.

Intradiscal electrothermal therapy (IDT) involves inserting a heating wire into the disc to strengthen the collagen fibers that hold the disc together.

Spinal fusion may be used to remove the injured disc and immobilize the spine around it.

Finally, disc replacement is possible. Here the disc is simply removed and replaced with a synthetic disc.

# Back Pain And Arthritis Of The Spine

Arthritis is inflammation of the joints. There are more than 100 rheumatic diseases and conditions that are types of arthritis. They affect joints, the tissues which surround the joints and other connective tissue. Arthritis is characterized by pain and stiffness in and around one or more joints. There are three main types of arthritis that affect the spine. They are osteoarthritis, rheumatoid arthritis and ankolyzing spondylitis.

Osteoarthritis is a disease in which the cartilage that cushions the ends of the bones at the joints wears away.

This causes the bones of the joint to rub together, causing pain, stiffness and bone spurs. The bone spurs can break off and float around in the joint, causing more damage and pain. The joint can become misshapen over time. Osteoarthritis is the most common form of arthritis. Osteoarthritis usually first strikes after the age of 40, and becomes more likely with age. People with osteoarthritis usually have joint pain and limited movement.

Rheumatoid arthritis occurs when the body's immune system attacks the tissue that lines the joints, the synovial membrane. White blood cells, the agents of the immune system, travel to the synovium and cause inflammation (synovitis). During the inflammation process, the normally thin synovium becomes thick and makes the joint swollen and puffy to the touch, leading to joint pain and inflammation. The inflamed synovium leads to erosion of the cartilage and bone within the joint. The muscles, ligaments and tendons around the joint weaken, and provide less support to the joint.

Rheumatoid arthritis is usually accompanied by fatigue and fevers. It usually begins in middle age and is more common in women than men.

Ankylosing spondylitis is a chronic form of arthritis that affects the spine and the sacroiliac joint, where the spine meets the pelvis. It can also affect the hips and shoulders. In severe cases, bone spurs form on the vertebrae. These can fuse the vertebrae together, causing the spine to become rigid, resulting in a great loss of mobility. Ankolyzing spondylitis is most often first diagnosed in young men, usually under the age of 35.

**How To Win Your War Against Back Pain**

Arthritis is typically treated with medication, either a pain reliever or an anti-inflammatory. Pain relievers include analgesic medications like aspirin and acetaminophen (Tylenol). Topical analgesics such as Zostrix, Icy Hot and Ben Gay can be effective in some cases where a pill-based medicine is not. NSAIDs, or non-steroidal anti-inflammatory drugs, are used to reduce swelling. These include such nonprescription medications as ibuprofen (Motrin, Advil), ketoprofen (Actron, Orudis) and naproxen sodium (Aleve).

Stronger prescription-based anti-inflammatories are available, including COX-2 inhibitors like celecoxib, which may be easier on the stomach than traditional NSAIDs.

Exercises will also be used to increase range of motion. These include various stretching and strengthening exercises to reduce the damage of the arthritis.

# <u>Massage Therapy And Back Pain</u>

A registered massage therapist is a trained in the assessment and diagnosis of injuries of the soft tissue and joints of the body. They use a blend of modern science and ancient philosophies to treat many conditions. A massage therapist has many potential treatments at their disposal. Massage therapy is becoming more widely accepted in the medical community as a credible treatment for many types of back pain. Studies have shown that massage therapy can benefit back pain sufferers by increasing blood flow and circulation, decreasing tension in the muscles, reducing pain caused by tight muscles and even improving sleep. Massage therapy can provide relief for many common conditions that cause back pain, such as arthritis, fibromyalgia, sports injuries and various other soft tissue sprains and strains.

Massage is non-invasive and considered very low risk for most people. In addition to physical benefits, massage is usually very relaxing. This can have profound psychologically benefits, particularly to someone suffering from chronic back pain. Depression is a symptom of chronic pain. Massage is thought to release endorphins, those natural chemical of the body that make you feel good and act as pain suppressors.

It is estimated that 75% of healthcare providers have sent patients of theirs to a massage therapist. If appropriate, you may want to ask your physician for a referral to a massage therapy professional in your area.

Most episodes of acute lower back pain are caused by muscle strain, such as from lifting a heavy object, or a traumatic injury like a sudden movement or a fall. The low back pain can be very severe and last anywhere from several hours to a couple of weeks. When back muscles are strained or torn, they can become inflamed.

With inflammation, the muscles in the back can spasm and cause both severe lower back pain and difficulty moving. Massage can help work out the spasm/irritation and improve range of motion. The large upper back muscles are also prone to irritation, either due to weakness or overuse.

Spinal arthritis is the inflammation of the joints of the spine. It can cause the breakdown of the

**How To Win Your War Against Back Pain**

cartilage between the aligning facet joints in the back portion of the spine. As the facet joints become inflamed they create frictional pain as bone rubs on bone. Therapeutic massage can help reduce osteoarthritis pain by improving circulation and reducing stress and muscle tension. However, it is important to find a professional who is specifically trained in treating people with arthritis.

Fibromyalgia is a widespread musculoskeletal pain and fatigue disorder for which the cause is still unknown.

Fibromyalgia means pain in the muscles, ligaments, and tendons, and is usually characterized by pain, stiffness and fatigue. The patient typically feels both widespread pain and pain in specific points as evidenced by physical examination. Massage can target both the tender points and the more broadly distributed pain and stiffness.

Although massage therapy is relatively safe, it is always advisable for patients to first check with their doctor before any treatment. Massage may not be suitable to those who have had recent surgery or who suffer from osteoporosis.

# Exercise For Back Pain

When you suffer from back pain, you are advised to handle it in a proper manner. When it is experienced, you must either lie down on bed or at least stop the stressful activity whichever you are performing currently.

Try to relax yourself completely as much as possible. If you have minor back pain, then it can be cured by taking rest for some time. But if still not cured, then you should be alert and careful to take proper steps to cure it fully.

The best solution is to do mild exercise for rehabilitating spine and curing the back pain from its root.

Exercise is the only proper way to heal completely from back pain. It is really hard to believe that by moving the part of your body which is paining can actually make you feel better. There are some specific exercises to strengthen your back and get relief from pain.

But yes! Take proper guidance before doing any major exercise. Consult your doctor or health care provider to see if exercise for back pain might be an option for you.

If so, the doctor may refer you to a physical therapist who will guide you through a specific exercise for back pain. Alternatively, your doctor or health care provider might be able to provide you with a list of specific exercises you can do on your own at home.

Sometimes back pain occurs due to lack of exercise.

This becomes very painful and occurs mainly in lower back when a person suddenly walks or stands for extended period of time. Then he/she thinks of not doing exercise.

Advantages of back exercise:
1) Discs get nutrition
2)  Builds and strengthens the back muscles
3)  Surgery Recovery faster

4)  Improves flexibility

Your exercise for back pain regimen might be one or a combination of stretching, strengthening or low-impact aerobic exercise. Low-impact aerobic exercise such as walking, bicycling and swimming has multiple health benefits in addition to potential for back pain relief.

Some specific back exercises

1)  Hip extension
2)  Stretches like pectoral stretch, lumbar side stretch, calf stretch
3)  Backward bending
4)  Press ups
5)  Dead lift

'Dead lift' is considered to be the best back exercise. Though it cures the back much faster than other exercises, it's not applicable for all as it requires more strength. It may even result to injuries if not undergone properly. This exercise must be done under the guidance of some exercise expert. Start from lifting the light weight and then go for heavy weights.

At last, finally comes the resting part, which is the most important part of exercise. Take complete rest to get better effect after doing your workouts. So start exercise from today and remain fit.

# Exercise For Back Pain: Using Golfers' Back Exercises

Back exercises go a long way in treating your back disorder. If you have ever played golf, you will realize how playing golf puts tremendous strain on your back creating back pain or a back injury.

Among the various back exercises 'golfer' is also included in the regular exercise discipline. It is necessary to understand the significance of the relieving effect of exercises on your back while playing golf.

A golf sway if clearly monitored, depicts clearly that the entire play is highly dependent on the extensive use of your back. A person having a back disorder would find it extremely difficult to play golf. Playing golf would be the most tedious task for him. Probably he might just succeed in playing the game. T

he extra efforts for the improvement of his golf game would be nearly impossible for him because of the acute back pain.

Golfers have to be extremely skillful in their game of golf. Back pain should not hinder their efforts in becoming a successful golfer.

It is advisable to go in for such exercises that would enhance the golfer's improvement in the game. The back exercises mentioned in 'Golfer' would come handy to a golfer having back pain. Golfers might develop a back problem due to the excessive usage of their back in playing golf.

These exercises would definitely give some remarkable relief from their back disorder and can guarantee their all round development in the game of golf.

Golfer's exercises can prove useful to them as golfers generally have a tendency to develop back pain as the back is put to maximum strain and use in the course of the game.

The game basically revolves around swaying your back to play the game and the resultant back injury cannot be avoided. Golfers with no history of back pain can stick to the exercise routine of

**How To Win Your War Against Back Pain**

'golfer' exercises to avoid any kind of discomfort to the back and play a healthy game of golf. People who have enrolled themselves in the 'golfer' exercise schedule have been lucky enough to get rid of the back pain altogether.

Some golfers though not entirely recovered have got a great amount of respite from back pain due to 'golfer' exercise method. This exercise would prove extremely beneficial for those who do not include exercise in their regular routine before playing golf.

People interested in the game of golf may retreat thinking that the game would prove more detrimental to their back. There is no need to be tense thinking the problems occurring to your back because of the game of golf.

Good players in the golf ground should enroll themselves in the 'golfer' exercise program and can rest assured regarding their back problems as 'golfer' would take care of the problem and make it disappear or reduce it to a minimal degree.

Play golf to your heart's content and enjoy the game with absolutely no hassles of back disorders with the aid of 'Golfer' exercise schedule.

# Exercise For Back Pain: Exercise Your Pain Away

Computer jobs are increasing and so are the back pain cases. According to the research done in foreign countries, it has been visualized that around 80% of people there will be suffering from the back pain.

If you have back pain, then take full rest and do light exercises which would help to stabilize spine. Do exercises which corrects muscle imbalance and makes muscles more flexible. It must be for core muscles, which are between shoulders and hips. The imbalances caused by these muscles causes back pain. The full stress comes on spine if the thighs back side is weaker than front.

This pain occurs due to following reasons:

1. Sitting or Standing for long time
2. Running for long distance
3. Vertebral Column sways back
4. Improper exercise of strength training

While doing any exercise related to strength training, deep breathing proves to be very effective. While pressing the leg toe, inhale deeply during bending and exhale during pressing. This proves to be very much helpful to increase length of spine and effectively utilizing the diaphragm muscles for supporting the spine.

**Exercises to reduce back pain:**

*1) The Tummy Tuck*

It is a simple pelvic move that brings the abdominal muscles up and away from floor. Relax for some time by keeping the face down on the floor and squeeze your buttocks to strengthen your spine. Reach your tail bone down towards the heels. Perform alternately for two sets each with twelve counts.

*2) The Bridge Lift*

This exercise is done by placing your feet on floor or a bench and scooping your pelvis in an upward motion. Your ribs should remain in lower position to reduce pull on your spinal muscles. Focus completely on muscle contraction.

### 3)  *The Lumbar Side Stretch*

This is done in standing and sitting position. While bending your knees, widen up your legs as much as possible. Now, put your one hand behind your head and bring the other hand down towards your feet on the inner side of thighs.

### 4)  *The Hip Flexor Stretch*

This is performed by bringing one foot ahead in an angle of 90 degree. The other leg is behind on floor with your foot pointed upwards. This exercise helps to extract muscles near hips on spine's side. You can squeeze your buttocks to feel stretch more. Stretching sensation must be experienced in back leg, front thigh and hamstrings of front leg.

### 5)  *The Calf Stretch*

This is intended to help strengthen the Achilles tendon. Put an object below your feet and lean whole weight of your body in a forward direction. Hold these stretches for 30 seconds and release. You will begin to feel a stretch on the back on the knee and shin area. Consult the Doctor and start exercise today.

# Exercise For Back Pain: 3 Types Of Exercises

Exercises are very much essential to keep our body fit. Three such types of exercises are shown here to reduce the lower back pain. You must have performed these exercises some time. But it is necessary to know exactly how to do the particular exercise. Yes, it's easy.

The following are three simple exercises which will help you to reduce back pain or any such recovery from injury.

## 1) Press-up

Through this exercise, you can relieve the stiffness from lower spine as well as hips. To do this exercise, lie down with face on floor. Put your both palms down and hands on sides of face. Press your shoulders and head upwards and rest on elbows. Hold your breath for 10 seconds and then release slowly. Then, rest completely on hands fully lifted so as to get more curve on lower side of your back. Perform three such sets.

## 2) Cat and Cow Pose

This exercise helps in stretching back so as to improve mobility. Keep your back flat and hands below shoulders. Spread the fingers and place the knees under the hips. Keeping your eyes closed, exhale and fold the back as a cat. Tuck your pelvis. Round up your shoulders. While lowering down your head, look at the knees. Keeping your eyes closed, concentrate on the movement of spine vertebrae and feel the stretch and contraction of muscles. Control properly the inhalation and exhalation. Bring head in upward position and slowly open eyes. Look forward and repeat this exercise for ten times. Better concentration will be more effective and also helps in preventing the injury in future also.

## 3) Hamstring Kick

This is helpful in stretching the hamstring as well as calf muscles. It also helps in getting relief from nerve pain. Lie down on the floor. Firstly, lift the right leg at 90 degree angle. With both hands, firmly hold thigh to lock up the leg in a stable position. In the same position, try to straighten up your leg. As soon as you feel the pull on the back side of the calf or knee, stop it. Hold it for ten seconds and slightly bend knee. Do the same with another leg.

These three exercises will be very much helpful and beneficial for lower back pain. Walking is

**How To Win Your War Against Back Pain**

also the best exercise. Start waling daily for 20-30 minutes and see the results. Walk straight and maintain your posture.

Tighten up your buttock muscles giving support to your back.

Thus, exercise for back pain need not be vigorous to be beneficial and your doctor is still the best judge. Just remember that simple exercises such as walking and stretching can have a huge impact on not only back pain, but aches and pains all over the body.

# Exercise For Back Pain: 3 Exercises For Sciatica

Do you feel pain or numbness in one side of the body or at the lower back area? It could be the symptoms of sciatica. Sciatica is a form of pain felt in the back area near the buttocks, legs or foot. Some people may also experience numbness, difficulty in leg and hip movements. But relax, the pain can be lessened or literally erased with three easy physical exercises.

Sciatica could be effectively eliminated from your body by following certain exercise forms.

Life could be so cheerful and relaxed without the constant pain of sciatica. You could walk all you want or play with kids or do anything you like without sciatica pain obstructing your every move.

If you are really serious about improving your health and quality of life, then just follow these simple exercises that may help eliminate sciatica:

*a.* ***Abdominal Area:*** The muscular abdominal region is one of the most vital muscles for the pelvic and spinal cord area. This muscle is main support system for the lower back area. Therefore to strengthen these muscles you need not do typical sit-ups, they may actually do more harm than good. If you help the abdominal muscles to get good amount of blood supply, then you require doing some muscle strengthening tactics such as the following:

*b.* ***Relaxing or easing your hip region:*** the hip muscle when in a tight position tends to amplify your pressure on the lower back region leading to a sciatica condition. Therefore to relax your hip muscles, you have to do some stretching exercises, you will feel the difference within a few days.

*c.* ***Piriformis Muscular Exercise:*** The Piriformis muscles are those next to the sciatic nerve. Therefore phirformis stretching exercises are important for prevention of sciatic pain. The work out is relatively easy to perform like the abdominal exercise.

The important point to note down while doing the stretch exercises is to know the correct method or knowledge of how or when to do it. This is the magic key to a pain free back or

**How To Win Your War Against Back Pain**

buttocks. The three most vital muscular regions are abdomen, hip flex, and piriformis.

If you mark these areas, which are main culprits for starting a sciatica pain, then you will soon get rid of the irritating pain.

Sciatica is a controllable ailment and you can win hands down with all the expert advice given in this article. You may have to learn few stretching techniques for the major muscular parts that act as a trigger for sciatica. When you accomplish to study them and act accordingly then be relieved that your sciatic pain is as good as gone.

# Exercise For Back Pain: Exercises For Post Partum Back Pain

Being pregnant and delivering a normal, healthy baby is a dream of every woman. But the after effects of this unique and wonderful experience can be a bit stressful if you do not take proper care of your precious body. Just out of a normal delivery, and suffering from a post-partum pain? It is normal to have post-partum backache, due to sudden weight loss of ten to eleven pounds. Most women suffer from post pregnancy back pains because of positional changes in the body.

As your body cannot adjust to the bodily changes overnight, it takes real effort on your part to gain that original figure you had before the onset of pregnancy. Reinstating the body parts such as the abdomen, pelvic region, back and spinal area is very important for eliminating any back and muscular pains. It is advisable for a just delivered mother to start a vigorous exercise regime after five to six weeks after delivery.

Physical activities such as jogging, lifting weights should is not recommended. But you may try walking; also stretchy workouts and light yogic postures may help. These light fitness workouts may help you to effectively handle post-partum backache.

You may start off with walking at a moderate pace. A nice stroll around your garden or the neighboring pathway for hour an hour daily is sufficient to start with, but you could increase the time and pace gradually as days go by. A good walk can tone-up your muscular parts and help you shed some of the "baby" fat of pregnancy.

And in turn assist you to fight off post-partum backache. Some exercises for boosting muscular joints in the hip, buttocks, thigh and spinal area like isometric workouts can also be effective in controlling post-partum back pains.

You may also try out some form of muscle strengthening isometric workouts for the abdomen, thigh, and back area. You can try squeezing your shoulders in unison and heaving your chest forward, hold this position for a few seconds, and then repeat it 8 to 10 times for 2 times a day.

Stretching exercises are also recommended for post pregnancy stage, take care that you do not

**How To Win Your War Against Back Pain**

stretch too much or the pelvic or spinal muscles may get damaged.

A post pregnancy stage is very fragile and delicate, do not do any exercise that will tear or damage ligaments in sensitive areas. Slow stretchy workouts are best, if you do for 20 to 25 seconds for 2 to 3 times in a day.

Doing these physical fitness workouts is a sure fire way to drive any back or muscular post-partum pain and get back to your original shape.

# Exercise For Back Pain: Can Exercise Stop Back Pain?

So back is paining badly and you want to do something about it. is there a way to stop the nagging pain. Now you may wonder whether there are any exercise regimes for an aching back? You may ask one and all for some tips on how to handle a nagging backache?

Some feel good bed rest may solve the problem, but no too much lying down or rest may actually aggravate the situation badly. Not more than a day or two should be spent in rest, followed by physical activities and workouts. A good back pain work out program may help the nutrients of the body to distribute itself to all the parts simultaneously such as spinal cord, muscular parts, ligaments, nervy areas and other joints of the body.

Stretching exercises will make your back more supple and strong. Actually rest could trigger major weakness and make the joints more stiff and unyielding.

Exercising at the right time will also eliminate the back pain forever and you would also be saved from a future backache. It would increase the immunity strength of the body.

But before you start a proper exercise course, it is advisable to take instructions from a medical expert. All and any type of work out cannot erase the persistent backache; it depends on the type and nature of the back pain. Some are caused due to spinal injury, then consulting an orthopedic doctor. Even though the main target area should be the back, but the whole body should be involved while doing an exercise.

You can very well stop a backache and lower the stressful effects of it by some exercises. They strengthen the abdomen region, spinal area and muscular gluteus. You can consult a physical trainer or therapist to do these particular exercises. Although the stretching workouts are relatively easy and you may do so on a routine basis, a proper strengthen work out may need you to take 2 to 3 days time gap after very session.

Workouts like lying flat on your back area on an open and flat ground, bending the knees and doing some breathing exercises. Then raise your head and shoulders away from the ground and holding the position for 2 to 3 seconds. You can do this 10 to 12 times in each session, if

**How To Win Your War Against Back Pain**

you feel discomfort, then stop the workout and do it in a slower pace. Likewise, lying on your stomach and keeping the chest level upfront with the help of your hands and raising your back level to a easy stretchy position may also provide relief.

But it is advisable to consult a good therapist or doctor before following an exercise program.

# Exercise For Back Pain: Adolescent Back Pain

Back pain is the most prevalent condition existing in the US. Back pain attacks everyone irrespective of age.

Young adults suffering from this chronic condition is on the increase. This article would brief you on the reasons for back problem and the solution to counter attack this problem.

It is really surprising that young bodies have to face this problem at so early an age. Young children are so engrossed in their routine way of life, their life being shuffled between home, school and several extracurricular activities that very little time is at their disposal to spend at home.

This has an adverse impact on their eating schedule. They often fill their tummies with the junk food available outside which results in unhealthy consumption of food and the resultant back pain. Junk food contains a high proportion of fat material, which makes you obese. Over weight children often complain of back problem. Your choice of food should enhance the strength of bones but children never bother to consume healthy food, which could make your bones strong and hence the back pain.

Exercise and its positive effects on your body cannot be disputed. In the earlier days children used to spend major part of their time playing outdoor games and this used to lead to perfect fitness regarding physical health.

Back pain was a rare occurrence. Now the advent of Internet and several interesting games on the video has depleted their interest in outdoor games. They prefer spending time on the computer.

Lack of proper physical exercise and continuity in same seating posture for a long period of time has consequently led to the rising back problem among adolescents. Outdoor playing canalizes the flow of oxygen to the blood in such a manner that they benefit your muscular cells and minimizes the chances of getting a back problem.

**How To Win Your War Against Back Pain**

The weight being borne by young people to their respective educational institutions enhances the back problem. Many a time they often carry games and clothes apart from the books.

This increases the burden on their back as their posture gets affected adversely due to the additional burden carried by them in back packs. A wrong notion is encouraged among children that all the items stuffed in a backpack are easy to carry whereas that is not very ideal for them.

This increased weight on their back consequently leads to severe back pain among young adults. Weak bones add to the severity of back pain.

In short young adults should go in for a perfect combination of food and exercise to keep them strong and healthy. Keep your bones strong by opting for a healthy style of eating and liberate yourself from the back problem that is constantly on the rise especially among young children.

# Exercise For Back Pain: Exercises To Do At Home

Exercise is the sure shot cure for majority of your health problems. Needless to say, this can cure your back problem also. Just to name a few, the below mentioned exercises will go a long way in healing your back pain. A brief consultation with the physiotherapist will start you on your way to a painless back.

- ***This exercise is beneficial for your abdominal muscles.*** Here you are expected to be in a lying posture with back touching the floor. Your feet should be kept flat touching the floor. Now bend your knees and then rise towards the ceiling. The next act is to reach your knees with your hands.

To do this move forward in such a fashion that your head and shoulders rise above the floor and then touch your knees. Remain in this posture for a count of 10. Then release yourself from this posture and relax. Repeat the above procedure for 5 times. This can guarantee the strength of your abdomen that supports your back.

- ***This exercise is directly related to back as you exercise your back more here.*** Place your hands on the hips in a standing posture with feet at a slight deviation from each other. Move your hand in a backward position such that it touches your back and keep your knees in a straight posture.

Now slowly bend backwards towards the waist but do not bend in such a manner that it enhances your back pain. Remain in this similar posture for 2 to 3 seconds and then come back to your normal position. The back muscles will be greatly benefited by this exercise and at the same time it will also loosen those muscles which are tight.

- ***You require a mat for this type of exercise.*** Lie with your face touching the floor and then try to lift one leg from the floor. The leg should remain in this rising position for a count of ten as this will stiffen the muscles in the leg also.

Then bring the leg back to the lowering position touching the floor. Try the same procedure with your other leg also. Keep this continued procedure for five more times and is sure to bring additional strength to your back muscles as well as your hip that supports your back.

***Warm up is quite mandatory before starting on any exercise.*** The best warm up for your body is walking. A back pain exercise require a certain amount of warm up before the actual exercise as this warm up decreases blood pressure, assure flow of blood to the heart and makes muscles more supple.

Heat up your body minutes before you start your back exercise and say a final goodbye to back pain.

# Exercise For Back Pain: Chronic Back Pain

Pleasure and pain are two sides of the same coin. Our experience with pleasure is quite memorable for us whereas our experience with pain leaves us bitter memories of the same. The intensity of pain varies from individual to individual.

Our way of handling pain is also of a different nature. One may have the capacity to bear the pain whereas the same pain can be intolerable to the other person. All of us experience toothache, headache, and several other painful ailments in our lives. Labor pain can be the most traumatizing for certain women. In short to handle pain is not an easy task and this article will advise you on how to handle chronic back problem.

The term chronic suggests that it has come to stay with us and back problem that stays with us throughout is difficult to deal with. The solution lies in the way the problem is dealt with. You can enter a phase of depression thinking about your pain and the amount of trouble it is causing you.

This can cause only harm to your body and mind as well. The best approach is to inculcate positive thoughts and register this fact in your mind that the pain is quite bearable and is not bothering you at all. But a person experiencing chronic back problem probably may not agree with you on this point saying that only the person undergoing the pain can know the trouble lying behind it.

But I would like to defer on this point. You are ultimately what your thoughts make you.

Exercise plays a dominant role in chronic back pain. Certain back exercises can stretch your muscles and this can prove to be an advantage to you as this enhances their strength.

A person having chronic back pain may find it a Herculean task to exercise as it causes pain to him.

Lack of exercise will only worsen the situation as the muscles become quite weak and then your slight movement can increase your pain. Chronic back pain should be handled in its initial

**How To Win Your War Against Back Pain**

stages and the person should click upon a solution to deal with his back problem.

Delays can increase your torture and make the pain unbearable. Your positive attitude towards life can help you take a step towards exercise and sort out many health problems.

Medicines usually go a long way in treating chronic back disorders. Pain killers relieve you of your pain but they also carry a certain amount of addiction with them.

Certain drugs should be consumed after much research on that particular medicine as you become immune to them and then the dosage of the medicine need to be increased to relieve you of pain. Stronger doses of any medicine can only carry an adverse impact with it on your body.

Drowsiness sets in and your active life is adversely affected by it. Eventually your functioning of the brain becomes slow. Accelerate your positive thinking process and get hold of the right medicines with no side effects and get relief from chronic back disorders.

# Chiropractic Care For Pregnant Patients

Contrary to popular belief, chiropractic adjustment is very useful to expectant mothers as it is for new mothers. There is not danger to expectant mothers or the unborn child if the patient undergoes chiropractic adjustment treatment. Pregnancy causes many changes to the body and displacement of joints is one of the changes a patient needs to put up with. These changes range from discomfort to very painful conditions and Chiropractic adjustment can bring a world of comfort to the patient.

The very process of chiropractic adjustment is surrounded by a world of myths especially when it comes to expectant mothers. When a person thinks of chiropractic adjustment the first thought that comes to their mind is the pain that is caused by the process of turning, twisting and snapping of the bones and joints. Many people also go to the extremes of explaining the process as one where the patient is lying on the therapy table with the therapist sitting on the patient and twisting the limbs out of place. Nothing can be further from the truth. Chiropractic therapy is something that can do a world of wonders to the expectant mother as well as the child.

There is absolutely no danger of contracting birth defects by undergoing chiropractic adjustment. There are many obvious benefits of the therapy and these benefits include controlling the feeling of nausea as well as relieving lower back pain, something that is experienced by all expectant mothers. Neck and joint pains are also greatly reduced by the therapy.

Chiropractic therapy for pregnant women is believed to be very as far as the labor and delivery is concerned. The therapy is known to reduce the labor time considerably and make the actual delivery quite painless. Many women believe that it was the therapy that caused them to avoid a cesarean section delivery by keeping the patient's musculoskeletal system by keeping the system in good medical health.

Chiropractors are very skillful when it comes to treating pregnant women. So, just to be on the safe side it is always better to do some research and find a chiropractor who specializes in treating pregnant women. The International Chiropractic Pediatric Association was founded by the late Larry Webster and is a good place to locate a skilled chiropractor. In fact, a Webster certified chiropractor is considered to be among the most skillful chiropractor.

# <u>Deciding If Chiropractic Care Is Appropriate For Arthritis</u>

If you have ever suffered from the painful condition of arthritis you will know what it is to experience relief from the painful spasms. And patients of arthritis are constantly searching for ways to relieve themselves from the painful grip of the disorder. Chiropractic adjustment is one very promising procedure that can bring a lot of relief to the condition and in a very short period of time too.

Apart from arthritis chiropractic therapy can be extremely useful for painful joint conditions as well. It is your family doctor who will suggest if chiropractic therapy is good for you or if it is suited for your condition. Medical advice is the first requirement before deciding undergoing any therapy and though there are many options for treatment of arthritis many patients who have undergone chiropractic therapy swear by the benefits of the treatment.

On the other hand there are people who definitely decide to stay away from the treatment just on the hear-say from other patients who have had bad experiences from the treatment. It all depends on the therapist. Chiropractic therapy or chiropractic adjustment is not such a painful procedure, which is contrary to popular belief. The loud snapping and popping of bones is not the sound of the bones breaking but the sound of the gas bubbles trapped inside the joints.

Chiropractic treatment is the closest one can come to arthritis treatment. Most of the time the pain from arthritis is so severe that medical intervention is inevitable, most of the time this medical treatment entails surgery. In such conditions chiropractic treatment might not be the best choice to alleviate the painful symptoms.

Now for some information on the economics of the treatment of Chiropractic care. It is not a pretty idea. Not as far as the US is concerned that is. However there are places other than the United States where you can find very skilled chiropractic therapists. The subcontinent is one such destination. So, before going in for the treatment you should be sure if your insurance policy covers the treatment. Many insurance companies cover the treatment if the patient decides to go abroad for the treatment where the costs are just a fraction of what it would cost in any European country, this is popularly called 'medical tourism'.

**How To Win Your War Against Back Pain**

So if and when you do decide to resort to the therapy, you should first take your doctor into confidence as well as the therapist. Giving them the right information is the first step to a successful process. It is also important that you understand that chiropractic adjustment is an alternative treatment for arthritis. A sad fact is that modern medicine does not consider chiropractic adjustment at par with the rest of the medical world. However, Chiropractic professionals are working hard to convince the 'disbelievers' of the power of the therapy and their efforts are fast catching on with the number of people flocking for the treatment the world over.

# Exercises For Lower Back Pain

If you want your back to get back the strength it had a few years ago and get the agility you had previous to your back pains you need to set up a regular exercise routine for yourself. Among the various exercise programs for lower back pain you should try a few f them and decide which one s the most appropriate for you. However, whichever exercise program you decide on you should first check with your health care professional before embarking on the program.

When you do start out to plan your lower back pain exercise program you should keep in mind that the exercises should be done 3 times a day for at least 10 minutes each and gradually move up to 15 minutes for each exercise period. The total daily exercise routine must be not be les than 30 minutes. When you start your exercise routine it must be in the presence or supervision of your orthopedic surgeon or physiotherapist just to ensure that you are carrying out the exercises correctly and in the proper posture, then when you are sure that you are doing it correctly and that the exercises are having a positive effect you can move out to ding them on your own.

When you set out on your lower back exercise therapy the chiropractic therapist will probably suggest the following exercise routine:

**Ankle pumps:**
You will be required to lie on your back with your legs straight and elevate your ankles slowly about 10 times.

**Heel slides:**
This is also done on your back with your legs straight and bring your knees up slowly with your feet flat on the ground – this is repeated about 20 times.

**Abdominal contraction:**
This is done lying on your back with your knees bent and your palms resting on your abdomen. Then you must raise your body from your shoulders without lifting your feet – this is repeated 20 times. Remember to hold your breath when you raise your body up, hold for 3 seconds then lower it down while you breathe out.

**How To Win Your War Against Back Pain**

**Straight leg arises:**

You must lie on your back with one leg straight and one leg bent at the knee. Tighten your stomach muscles and hold your breath then raise the straight leg about 12 inches, hold for 3 seconds then relax. Repeat 20 times with each leg.

**Heel raises:**

Standing with your pals against the wall you must raise your heels up by standing on your toes. Breathe in while you raise yourself up. Hold for 5 seconds then relax. Repeat 20 times.

**Wall squats:**

Finally the last exercise will be the wall squats. Keep your back against a wall and slide your feet about a feet away from the wall. Keeping your abdominal muscles tight you should slide your body to a squatting position, without actually going all the way down. Hold this position for 5 seconds then stand up again. Repeat 10 times.

After doing these exercises for a week you will definitely find a great change in your lower back and will be able to lead a normal life. However, these exercise routine should be continued with to avoid getting back into the painful situation you have managed to get out of.

# Exercises For Sciatica

Patients of sciatica will definitely benefit form exercises that are scientifically researched and are known to provide relief in a short period of time. Different cases of sciatica call for different exercises and exercise routines and all the exercises must be done under supervision and done correctly or the patient will end up doing more harm than good.

Sciatica is a condition of the bone and can occur due to spinal stenosis brought on by herniated spinal disk or what is known as ' periformis' syndrome. The pain caused due to this condition may be felt in the lower back, thigh, foot, leg or the buttocks. Each symptom requires a different set of exercises and a regime that must be adhered to religiously if relief must be attained and sustained.

Some of the best exercises for sciatica will move the pain from the lower extremities back up to the lower back where the pain is then cured or contained in a more bearable limit. Press-up r extension exercises have been known to work well for the symptoms of sciatica.

In the most effective exercise for sciatica the patient is required to lie on his or her back and prop the upper body up on the elbows. The hips of the patient must be flat on the floor. Remember that this exercise is done on the hard surface of the floor and not on a cushioned surface. Lie in this position for 5 seconds the first day then slowly extend this position to 30 seconds. When the patient is comfortable doing this exercise it may be repeated 20 times daily. Raising the upper body on to the elbows with the forearms flat on the ground and holding for 30 seconds then lying down and relaxing. This exercise is repeated 20 times daily.

When this symptom is caused by spinal stenosis the best and most effective exercise is stretching. The patient needs to lie on his or her back with knees pulled up to the chest. The knees must be pulled as far up as possible until the patient feels a slight stretch without any discomfort. Hold this stretch for at least 4 seconds with a deep breath then lower the legs and relax for 10 seconds. Repeat this exercise at least 10 times daily.

Another exercise that strengthens the back and relieves sciatica is done lying on the back pressing the lower back to the floor by simply contracting the back muscles and relaxing them.

**How To Win Your War Against Back Pain**

Contract the lower back muscles along with the abdominal muscles and old this position for at least 5 seconds and then relax. Repeat this exercise 10 times.

A good stretching exercise for sciatica caused by piriformis syndrome is the patient lying on their back with the legs flat on the floor. Pull the painful leg towards the chest, while holding the knee on the same side and holding the ankle with the other hand. Try to pull the knee in the direction of the other ankle until you can feel the stretch. Do not try to force it beyond this point, but hold it for up to 30 seconds. Release it and start again, doing this three times.

These exercises are just a few of the many stretching and strengthening exercises that are helpful in relieving the pain caused by sciatica. A physical therapist, spinal specialist or chiropractor will be able to give the patient an entire list of different exercises.

# Lidocaine For Back Pain Relief – Is It Safe?

Sometimes known as Lignocaine, Lidocaine is a compound that is widely known as a good treatment for back pain relief. This is a local anesthetic and is also used as an anesthetic for insignificant surgeries and also for dental surgeries. This application for lower back pain is available in patches that can be applied on the skin. This patch contains only 5% Lidocaine and is known to always show positive results though the duration of the relief varied greatly and depends from patient to patient.

Patients of arthritis have been extensively treated with Lidocaine and have shown positive results with little of no side effects. Lidocaine works by blocking the pain signals at the nerve endings and numb the nerves blocking all pain signals to the brain. This is very effective treatment especially for patients suffering from arthritis.

There are reports from various quarters about the side effects of the treatment, however, there are more reports of the good and effective points of this treatment as compared to the adverse reports of the treatment, which, we may add are directed towards the misuse of the treatment. Another reason for the controversy may be because the treatment is not approved by the FDA. However, the medical fraternity is waiting patiently because the approval may come sooner than expected and with it a lot of patients will be relieved of their lower back pain.

One ore method of administration of Lidocaine is through injections directly into the back. This treatment lasts for just a couple of hours and so is rarely used except in dire emergencies. This treatment is mostly used to confirm a diagnosis and for locating the exact muscle that is causing the problem. The fast acting ingredient is best suited for arriving at a diagnosis and deciding on the treatment for the painful condition.

There are a lot of products on the market with Lidocaine as the main ingredient for pain relief. Many of these products are roll on types and are very effective in treating the symptoms of back pain. However, before buying over the counter lidocaine applications you should have a discussion with the pharmacist as to which applicant is best suited for your needs.

**How To Win Your War Against Back Pain**

With the imminent approval of the FDA for the use of Lidocaine as a pain reliever in cases of arthritis and lower back pain symptoms, people are beginning to gain confidence in the medication that has been engulfed in controversy over the past few years. Lidocaine is not a cure for pain but just a temporary relief from pain while the physicians try to locate the cause of the pain. And until then they can resort to the use of Lidocaine containing applicants to relieve the pain while the treatment continues and a permanent cure is achieved over a period of time.

# Lower Back Pain With Stomach Pain

Having to bear lower back pain accompanied with stomach pain is an experience no one should ever have to go through. Scientists and doctors all over the world are groping around, mostly in the dark, trying to put their finger on the cause of lower back pain. So far as women are concerned doctors are sure that lower back pain accompanied with stomach pain is related to their menstrual cycles and this is something that can be dealt with a fair amount of ease.

However, doctors have admitted that it is not an easy thing to pinpoint the cause of lower back pain accompanied with stomach pain. They insist that a patient who can keep a track of the symptoms and report them to the doctor will make the process of diagnosing the cause and arriving at a better and effective treatment an easier task.

Some of the causes of lower back pain accompanied with stomach pain are related to the more common urinary infections and kidney or bladder problems, then again you may have a serious bowel problem. Whatever the cause of your lower back pain and abdominal pain you will soon find that it is very difficult to pinpoint and even more difficult to treat effectively. Most treatments available will prove to be temporary in nature and the condition will recur frequently.

In most cases where the lower back pain is caused by a urinary tract infection or cystitis a bout of stomach pain is also accompanied along with the lower back pain. There will also be a bit of inflammation in the abdominal region. There will mostly be a burning sensation in the stomach or back. Kidney stones are another reason for lower back pain and stomach pain.

If lower back pain accompanied by stomach pain is caused by kidney stones the pain will be so severe that the patient will not be able to stand or sit. In such cases the best resort is to use a local anesthetic to relieve the pain temporarily while the doctor treats the cause of the pain. In more unfortunate cases the pain is caused by tumors in the kidney and this scenario will have to be dealt with by the best experts in the field. Self, over the counter medication is strictly ruled out in cases where the pain is caused by kidney malfunctions or dysfunctions.

Doctors may also consider dysfunctions of the bowels to try to locate the cause of lower back pains accompanied by stomach pains. In such cases the doctor may prescribe some pathological tests to arrive at the proper conclusion and also to decide which medication is the best suited for the patient's recovery. One sure-shot way to tell if the back pains and stomach pains is caused by the bowels is that the pain will come in waves, mostly between small amounts of exertions. Remember to tell the doctor this if he does not ask. Most lower back pains are cased by bowel disorders.

Other areas that your doctor will consider are the bowels. For instance both constipation and diarrhea can be painful. The doctor will do more tests if you indicate you've had a change in your bowel patterns when you began to get lower back pain with stomach pain. One surefire way to tell if you are experiencing pain from the bowels is the nature of the pain itself. It would come in waves with minimal discomfort, or none at all in between the pain.

If you happen to have lower a bloated or swollen lower belly, this may be a warning flag for conditions such as irritable bowel syndrome. Notice fresh blood or tarry looking stools? This would need investigating as well.

Your pain may feel like it's coming from the womb or any other of your internal reproductive organs. This would mean you would experience the pain in the middle of the lower belly, just above the line of public hair about as far up as the navel. There might be more pain to one side than the other – usually an indication of an ovary being inflamed etc.  If you have pain when you have sex, you would feel that deep in your pelvic area. The possible range of conditions is varied. You could be looking at pelvic inflammatory disease, ovarian cysts, fibroids or maybe even endometriosis. In any event, don't wait call your doctor immediately.

# <u>Non-Surgical Treatment For Chronic Back Pain</u>

Chronic back pain is a repeated condition that affects many people worldwide every year, but the cause of the complaint differs from person to person. At times, back pain may occur because the person has been in an accident or put undue stress on his or her back, pulled a muscle during exercising or regular chores or even slept on an uncomfortable surface etc. and this has resulted in a chronic condition for them.

The first step to studying treatment options open to persons suffering from chronic complaints for back pain is to begin looking back at what could have led to the condition: e.g. rewind to the possible causes so the treatment mode can be decided as this depends on what has caused the problem.

If it is some unknown reason, the pain is no less, but compounded with the doubt as to the cause of the back pain condition and so picking and choosing from the different types of back pain treatment options becomes all the more stressful for them. For severe cases of chronic back pain, medical health practitioners offer surgical treatment choice, but for moderate cases and even for those who fear going under the knife, there is no dearth of non-surgical treatments, such as inversion therapy and acupressure etc.

Many a time it is the patients that prefer to understand and explore the choices for non-surgical treatment options for chronic back pain, but it is not uncommon to find even doctors recommending non-surgical treatment for the same. Most ethical health practitioners will not recommend surgery to treat chronic back pain if there is another healthy and safe choice.

Suppose there is a very painful back problem, then medical specialists suggest to the patient's family to explore the option of surgery, especially if the condition can worsen without treatment or due to any delay in beginning some curative procedure e.g. in the case of the patient having degenerative spondylolisthesis or severe sciatica. At times, even in the above mentioned scenario, it has been known that non-surgical treatment for the condition has helped bring fast relief, but for complete relief, surgery is usually the best alternative.

**How To Win Your War Against Back Pain**

At other times, surgery may be necessary for the patient to perform all bodily functions properly in a normal manner, but if there are not too many limitations on the patient's lifestyle due to the back-paint, then other alternative therapies are preferred by both patient and doctor.

Some of these non-surgical treatments for back-pain include conservative techniques so as to rule out cancer (of the spine etc.), infection or an emergency medical issue due to injury and can be carried out best through heat therapy and taking adequate rest.

Non-prescription medications like ointments, balms, muscle relief sprays and roll-ons are also effective for back pain treatment and give immediate, fast relief often, especially when combined with heat-application therapy and rest.

Since chronic is a condition labeled so only if the patient has suffered it for a few months and the doctor has declared it so on examination, there may be cause for undertaking still other treatment options beyond the scope of applying heat, rest and pain relievers as effective techniques and physical therapy for treating injuries may also be put into application for the patient by a trained physiotherapist. Such a professional will guide the patient about the various ways in which to work the human body and teach them how to respond to certain situations.

# <u>Sciatica Treatment – Get It Done Early For Best Results!</u>

Chronic back pain is a terrible condition to suffer from and thousands of people all over the world have this complaint, but for it to be considered so, it has to be tagged by a medical expert after examination of the patient who should have had the complaint for at least a few months. Degenerative spondylolisthesis is one of the forms of chronic back pain while severe sciatica is the other very painful and trying type of back pain condition one can have.

In most of the cases, the complaint of sciatica heals on its own, though it may take a few days and at the most a week or so. In other cases, the person suffering from sciatica back pain may complain of having severe bouts of pain or even frequent occurrences of back pain episode flaring up, which may seem unbearable but are actually a warning sign to the patient to get immediate treatment carried out.

If the patient finds that these recurring flare-ups of sciatic back pain are more frequent than usual, then he or she must take it as a sign for consulting a medical expert for exploring the various options for initiating proper treatment for their specific condition i.e. sciatica pain.

In order to understand what sciatica pain is, in simple terms, it can be defined as a dull to throbbing pain that originates from the sciatic nerve, rising in intensity if not attended to; in severe cases, it is recommended that treatment be started immediately.

Depending on what stage of sciatica back pain the patient is at, simple and regular physical exercise regimes may be developed and followed by the person under the guidance of a professional physiotherapist, medical doctor or personal trainer who also has knowledge of pain management methods so these can be quickly and effective put into service as and when the patient needs them.

If the sciatica back pain is very severe and the case cannot be helped even with over the counter medication combined with regular exercise programs, then the patient must be guided towards considering more advanced levels of physical therapy, other non-invasive procedures of treatment, alternative therapies such as acupuncture and acupressure before taking the ultimate step of back pain surgery.

**How To Win Your War Against Back Pain**

However, what often happens is that people are scared of going under the knife and actively avoid surgery even when it can be good for them in the long run; such patients must be counseled about the merits of the sciatica surgery and made to understand to what extent the quality of their life can be improved if they opt for proper treatment, including surgery.

Once the exact cause of the sciatica pain has been determined, the doctor can work towards explaining the various techniques that are most useful and effective in treating the condition; this typically includes hot and cold fermentations for the back as well as the legs in the initial stages of the disorder, beginning with only 20 minutes at a stretch 4-6 times a day.

Other treatment options for sciatica patients include taking non-prescription anti-inflammatory medication like ibuprofen, or taking the recourse of having an epidural steroid injection administered to them, both of which help reducing and ultimately relieving the pain and inflammation. Injections for treating sciatica pain are more effective though, as they are delivered to the specific area of the pain and work immediately as compared to the pills; they can be safely expected to work for up to a year.

# Possible Causes For Sharp Lower Back Pain

In this article, we take a look at the importance of learning the causes of lower back pain, especially if it a sharp shooting kind of pain and determining the causes of origin of the pain. So, if you are truly feeling laid-back in the literal sense of the word and have suffered sharp lower back pain more than once recently, perhaps its time to do some quick thinking about what could have brought it on – so you can begin the right course of treatment based on the diagnosis, which needs to be proper and accurate.

Only after a proper medical examination of the person's past activities, especially ones involving heavy physical labor, can a person's cause for personal back pain due to injury or other reasons be pinned down accurately. Among the most common reasons triggering off lower back pain are sudden exertion, carrying heavy loads, standing, sitting or lying down in an awkward posture (e.g. such as painting the ceiling with a hand overhead all the time) and bending or twisting in a casual, thoughtless manner – which can happen during exercising as well as during regular household chores.

Sharp lower back pain can also become a chronic condition if not addressed in the initial stages and therefore doctors and medical health experts, including physical trainers and gym instructors advise people against exercising too much or wrongly, without proper knowledge of the right techniques since twisting wrong and doing heavy physical work can also aggravate a mild condition. Sometimes, patients tend to ignore the initial warning signs of a sharp lower back pain thinking it will go away and its not worth bothering over, but this is wrong and needs to be addressed immediately to prevent more severe cases. What many do not realize is that in ignoring the warning signal given by the body to the individual, there is a chance of aggravating an already painful condition and therefore, patient information on the condition is very crucial to serve a timely warning.

If the patient does not recall any of the above scenarios as causes for the lower back pain he or she is suffering, medical opinion should be sought immediately to rule out other possibilities, such as conditions of spinal stenosis (restricted spinal cord and nerve root channels), arthritis, infection in the spine, cancer of the spine or spondylolisthesis.

**How To Win Your War Against Back Pain**

Also, a doctor is the best person to rule out the possibility of a fracture in the lower back as a potential cause for the sharp pain a patient may be suffering; once the above possibilities have been studied and other acute or chronic areas of the condition have been looked into, then diagnosis is more likely to be accurate and treatment can be started in earnest.

Some of the signs that a lower back pain sufferer may need to put across to his or her doctor for proper diagnosis include a sort of general ache radiating into the lower back, behind and the legs with occasional or steady complaints of numbness, tingling or weakness. Those suffering additional bowel or bladder problems should not delay contacting their doctor as this could mean a more severe case of lower back pain than usual.

Examination of the condition typically includes slow and careful palpation of the spine to determine nature of muscle spasms, displacements/sore points and the same is also carried out for the abdomen to verify the involvement of any organ in the complaint. To determine the exact origin of sharp lower back pain, doctors may also recommend the patient undergoing neurological assessments, lab tests and imaging studies.

How To Win Your War Against Back Pain


This Product Is Brought To You By


# DAVID A OSEI

www.ingramcontent.com/pod-product-compliance
Lightning Source LLC
Chambersburg PA
CBHW031244250726
48655CB00005B/2075